Contents

THE SECRET TO BEING THIN

EAT 6X A DAY EVERY 2½ HOURS FROM THE LIST

MacroWise

ISBN: 979-8-9898200-3-0
Independently published.

PREFACE

By Asher

*"I have put before you, life, and death. . .
choose life so that you may live."*

-Deuteronomy 30:19

Some of the greatest challenges in life often have very simple solutions. I was a drug addict for 15 years and couldn't get clean no matter how many times I tried. I sought help from the best doctors, detox clinics, rehab centers, hypnotherapists, peer-support groups, etc., and none of it made a difference. I always ended up relapsing just as soon as the physical pain and mental cravings kicked in. The hardest part about breaking any addiction is overcoming the withdrawal symptoms. I knew there had to be some healthy, natural substance I could take to keep me satisfied while getting off drugs. Once I found a simple method to ease my pain and nullify my cravings, I stopped using drugs and stayed clean permanently.

Throughout those 15 years as a drug addict, I developed a very bad habit of eating whatever I wanted whenever I felt like it. After I got clean, it became clear to me that I was grossly overweight and out of shape. So, I made the decision to lose weight and get fit, which led me to find a plan. I knew there were tasty, natural foods I could eat instead of junk to stay satisfied. I took the same approach I used for getting off drugs and applied it to losing weight. Once I found a simple method to satisfy my hunger and nullify my cravings, I stopped eating junk food and lost weight permanently. After helping other people do the same, I knew this natural replacement method could work for anyone, which is why I created MacroWise.

I'm not a doctor, scientist, or registered dietitian, but I've gained real experience through overcoming drug and sugar addiction. And I guarantee you that sugar is a highly addictive, dangerous drug that's responsible for a worldwide epidemic of sick, fat people. In the United States, 42% of adults have obesity, and 1 out of 11 adults have severe obesity. Obesity is a leading cause of preventable death in the U.S. The main point you need to know is that an overweight person trying to lose weight can't eat sugary foods and expect to be thin. Just like a recovering cocaine addict can't use their drug and expect to maintain their sobriety. In both cases, the addict's occasional use of drugs fuels a vicious cycle of relapse and addiction.

MacroWise makes it easy to change the way you eat and lose weight permanently. Simply eat 6 times a day every 2 ½ hours from "the list" and follow the basic rules. This proven method is your solution for replacing bad with good and choosing life.

Part 1

MacroWise Lifestyle Program
*Book & coaching services are available
at MacroWise.com*

CHAPTER ONE

My Story — How MacroWise Was Born

I was 60 pounds overweight and wanted it gone. I was getting older and knew it was now or never. I decided to lose the weight but didn't have a good plan for doing it. I used to exercise a lot when I was younger, so I had an idea of what to do next. I started eating healthier foods and walking at night when it was cooler outside. That led to training with resistance bands at home, and eventually, I joined a gym. I was toning up but not losing any real body weight. It took me 3 months to lose 10 pounds doing it my way.

A few months into my weight-loss journey, my sister told me about a "macro-diet" she recently used to lose weight and began helping others do the same as a coach. She explained how you lose body fat by eating low-sugar, low-calorie foods, with a specific number of proteins, carbs, and fat, 6 times a day every 2 ½ hours without exercising. So, instead of eating whatever I wanted and whenever I felt like it, I would eat their portion-controlled, macro-friendly snacks 5X a day plus 1 meal with protein & vegetables. She promised that if I followed the plan by only eating the foods from their list, I would never be hungry, and the fat would come right off. Even though the diet seemed overly strict and their snacks contained unhealthy ingredients, I decided to go with it. The first few days were the hardest because of the withdrawal symptoms from sugar detox, but I followed the plan and consistently lost 2 ½ pounds each week. After 6 weeks, I started to look and feel better, but I was sick of eating their foods and getting tired of the diet.

During those 6 weeks, I learned how to read food labels and understand the number of calories and the ratio of macronutrients I needed per serving to lose weight. I searched online at Amazon and scoured local grocery store shelves for better-tasting, natural snack options with the right number of calories, protein, carbohydrates, and fat. After 2 months on my sister's macro diet, I replaced all the old, stale, ultra-processed snacks from her inferior diet food company with new, fresh, wise-processed snacks from dozens of superior food companies. I replaced unhealthy, unnatural, un-savory, soy protein snacks, with healthy, natural, delicious, and nutritious protein snacks. I also found a variety of tasty, low-sugar marinades, sauces, condiments, and sides, that made every meal a pleasure. After transition-ing into "my-macro plan", I continued to lose 2 ½ pounds every week until reaching my goal weight. I lost 50 pounds in 6 months and kept it off for good. I would have lost twice the amount of weight in twice the time if I had more fat to lose. But 50 pounds was my number, so I stopped trying to lose weight at this point. Instead, I shifted my focus to maintaining my goal weight and getting lean.

The only week I didn't lose weight during that time was when I got drunk one night at a party and ate a bunch of junk food. Alcohol is something my sister made clear from the start to avoid while trying to lose weight. Alco-hol is considered the 4th macronutrient and contains 7 calories per gram, which is almost twice as many calories as a gram of protein. But unlike the 3 main macros - protein, carbohydrates, and fat, alcohol has no nutri-tional value. In addition to being high in empty calories, it stops the body from burning fat, can make you feel hungry, and leads to poor food choices. Avoiding alcohol was very helpful in reaching my goal weight quickly and maintaining it consistently.

So, after maintaining my goal body weight for 2 years and helping oth-ers lose weight too, I became convinced that I found the modern-day se-cret to being thin. Unlike restrictive diets such as keto, Atkins, Optavia, Nutrisystem, or my sister's macro diet, my macro plan was more flexible in allowing you to eat a variety of natural foods that contain more carbo-hydrates and tasty, healthy ingredients. I put together a list of snacks and essential groceries that have a macro-friendly ratio of protein, carbs, and fat and that keep you in your macro range and burn body fat. The list delivers hundreds of tasty, healthy, nutritious options to enjoy, so there's always something to look forward to. With my macro plan, you know exactly what and when to eat throughout the day, whether you're at home, at work, or dining out at a restaurant. You're never hungry until it's time to eat, and your new, skinny clothes always fit. Plus, you save a lot of time, money, and effort, since macro-friendly snacks are fast, inexpensive, and convenient to eat anytime, anywhere. Once I found the secret to being thin, I named it "MacroWise", for good reason, and wanted to share it with others in need of help.

During the first 2 years I maintained my goal weight, various people who witnessed my body transformation asked me for help, which is how I became a weight-loss coach. I explained that there are 2 basic rules for losing weight and keeping it off. Simply eat 6 times a day every 2 ½ hours from my curated list and stay within a specific calorie and macro range. They made adjustments to their lifestyles and got results. I coached them over the phone from time-to-time and exchanged text messages whenever they had basic questions. I started coaching more people after that for free because I truly care about others. Plus, I knew I could help them. The number of people asking for my list grew, along with the number of phone calls and text messages I was receiving for coaching. Around that time, a few of my successful clients expressed interest in taking some of those calls and texts, so they could help coach people too. They were hoping to get paid for their time, considering time is money and helping others requires a lot of it. I found that people were willing to pay for coaching when getting help from someone with real, first-hand experience. So, I hired the best people for the job, trained them, and began charging for the coaching service.

At that point, I decided the best way to help more people was to write this book and name it *The Secret to Being Thin*. I built a website to post my curated list of foods and drinks, along with active links to locate and purchase them. MacroWise became a real business once this book was released to the public. After that, the demand for coaching increased, as more and more people bought the book. Some people required more help than others and not everyone had the money to pay. That's when I decided to record a library of daily instructional videos to help people online, and I developed a network of live coaches to help over the phone. Creating smart coaching options provided an easy and affordable solution to anyone seeking help. Not everybody who buys this book needs coaching, and many do fine without it. This book is a proven manual for making simple adjustments to your life, so you can lose weight and keep it off.

Whenever someone asks me how much it costs to get MacroWise, I tell them it's free. It doesn't cost you any extra money to make the change. The food costs about the same and you can be successful without help from a coach. The only cost is if you paid for this book, but that's free too. Even better than free, this book offers you an opportunity to make money. If you follow the book as your manual and remain persistent, you will be successful. Send me before-and-after photos that show your success along with a receipt for this book, and I'll pay you $100. Plus, the photos can serve as your application to make more money while helping others as a MacroWise coach yourself. The gig pays generously and lets you set your own hours while working from home. Having a simple weight-loss plan that works combined with recruiting coaches from within is how MacroWise was born. You have nothing to lose and everything to gain by believing in yourself and making the decision to change.

There are plenty of other weight-loss programs that work well short-term if you exercise like an Olympian or only eat "their foods." The problem is that neither is sustainable. Very few people can commit to intense, regular exercise, which is not a solution on its own. Physical exercise will tone your body and clear your mind but does little to help you lose weight long-term. It's just a matter of time before an injury occurs or life gets in the way and it becomes difficult to exercise regularly. And staying devoted to eating unsatisfying foods that are manufactured by profit-hungry, diet-food companies, isn't realistic either. Unfortunately, most of the foods that diets require you to eat are full of bad chemicals, too expensive, or hard to follow. These are common examples of how so many people start a weight loss program, lose some weight, and then quickly relapse, only to gain it all back again.

There are two ways to get where you want to be in life. There's the "short-long" way and the "long-short" way. You can take shortcuts to lose weight, like fad diets, fasting, and diet drugs, to reach your goal weight quicker, but the results don't last and it takes longer to achieve your goal over time. Or you can go the long-short way, which appears to take longer at first. But once you reach your goal weight, it sticks! When it comes to losing weight, MacroWise is the way to get where you want to be in life and keep you there for good. 80% of what you eat determines how you look and feel, which means you really are what you eat. If you want to be thin and feel good permanently, then MacroWise is the answer.

To be clear, MacroWise was not created to profit from your personal struggles in life. All the foods, drinks, supplements, and other items we recommend are sold by 3rd party, independent companies. MacroWise provides a plan for losing weight, the support to actualize it, and a list of foods to sustain it. Eating the tasty, nutrient-dense foods on the list 6 times a day every 2 ½ hours is the secret to being thin.

MacroWise was born out of a desire to share knowledge with others in need of help. Just like my sister lost weight and coached me, I followed by helping others, and now you can do the same. This circle of life relationship is founded on giving, receiving, and healing. Passing down this knowledge to anyone in need of help is a great honor and privilege.

Welcome to MacroWise!

CHAPTER TWO

What Is MacroWise?

There are many diet plans, such as keto, Atkins, Optavia, and Nutrisystem, that can help you lose weight short-term but fail to be sustainable for most people long term. They involve tweaking, tracking, and regulating the calories, macros, and foods you consume. Almost all calories come from 3 macronutrients - protein, carbohydrates, and fat. Each macro provides a different calorie amount per gram. 1 gram of protein contains 4 calories, 1 gram of carbohydrates contains 4 calories, and 1 gram of fat contains 9 calories. Your daily calorie and macronutrient intake consists of the total number of protein, carbs, and fat, you consume each day.

Diet plans, like keto and Atkins, require a major increase in fat intake and a significant reduction of carbohydrates. While other diets, like Optavia and WonderSlim, focus on low-fat intake and allow moderate carbohydrates. Tweaking your calorie intake and macro ratio can put your metabolism into fat-burning mode, which is a fast and effective way to lose weight. Unfortunately, both high-fat and low-fat diets are unhealthy long-term, which makes them unsustainable. Plus, they typically require you to invest a lot of time, effort, and discipline into planning, grocery shopping, and making your own food. Unless you have lots of free time or a personal chef, it's not likely you will stay committed to a restrictive diet. There are also plenty of easy diet plans, like Nutrisystem and Jenny Craig, that you can follow as well, but they require you to only eat their prepared foods, which is boring and hard to stomach long-term. Most diets eventually lead to regression into old eating habits, relapse, and weight gain. The truth is, if a person is unable to adopt a better way of eating for life, then their weight loss is almost always temporary.

For people who like the short-term results of diets like keto, Atkins, Paleo, Optavia, and Nutrisystem but don't like the strict rules of any diet long-term, then MacroWise is the answer. MacroWise is a simple lifestyle that embraces proven principles found in other weight-loss programs and rejects the annoying details responsible for the high dropout rates. With MacroWise, you get to eat 6X a day every 2 ½ hours without exercising. You're allowed to have triple the amount of carbohydrates than keto. You get access to a vast, curated list of tasty, nutrient-dense foods, supplied by hundreds of vetted, high-quality food companies. And there's an amazing variety of delicious, naturally sweet desserts you get to enjoy. The macro-friendly foods on the list contain the right number of calories and macronutrients needed to satiate your appetite, crush your cravings, and burn your fat. Having access to an extensive list of macro-wise foods you love, makes it easy to stick to the plan long-term because you never get bored.

"The list" introduces you to a world of high-protein, low-carb, macro-friendly snacks called MacroWise snacks. "MacroWise snacks" are a fast, tasty, and convenient way to get the calories and macronutrients you need throughout your waking hours to stay satisfied and lose weight. There are hundreds of high-quality, pre-packaged, portion-controlled MacroWise snacks available online at Amazon. And there are countless, fresh whole foods you can buy at the grocery store for making your own snacks and meals at home. Keeping your kitchen stocked with tasty, macro-wise foods is essential for staying in your macro range and losing weight permanently. Eating the foods on the MacroWise list 6X a day every 2 ½ hours is the secret to being thin. This simple lifestyle saves you a lot of time, effort, and aggravation, from worrying about what, when, and where to eat. Plus, it helps you develop healthy eating habits you own for life.

Plenty of diet plans will tell you how to lose weight, but very few provide a realistic way to maintain your weight beyond that. MacroWise is a progressive lifestyle program comprised of 3 phases that provide a simple solution for being thin, lean, and healthy. The lifestyle begins with losing weight, before helping you get in shape and live a healthy life. For the first phase, it's necessary to kickstart your metabolism for up to 90 days by eating 5 MacroWise snacks plus 1 MacroWise meal with protein & vegetables each day. The "5 & 1-Thin Phase" focuses on rapid weight loss, which includes detoxing your brain and body from sugar by changing the way you eat. Your calorie intake should be between 1,000 to 1,300 per day, consisting of 100-125 grams of protein, 50-100 grams of carbohydrates, and 25-75 grams of fat. This calorie deficit and macronutrient ratio puts your body into fat-burning mode, which causes you to lose weight fast. Having a list of tasty, macro-wise foods is essential for making this key change.

After the 90-day Thin Phase is complete, you transition into the second phase, which is less restrictive. This is where you eat 4 MacroWise snacks plus 2 MacroWise meals a day. The "4 & 2-Lean Phase" focuses on losing weight at a slower but steady pace, since your calorie and macro allowance increases. Your calorie intake should be between 1,300 to 1,700 per day, consisting of 100-150 grams of protein, 75-125 grams of carbohydrates, and 50-100 grams of fat. This second phase opens the door to a wonderful, new variety of nutrient-dense foods, refreshing beverages, and naturally sweet desserts, all of which you can find on the list. Eating these foods 6 times a day every 2 ½ hours and completing some light exercise workouts is how you get lean and reach your goal weight.

After reaching your goal weight, you transition into the third and final phase where you get to enjoy a healthy balance of 3 MacroWise snacks plus 3 MacroWise meals a day. The "3 & 3-Healthy Phase" focuses on maintaining your goal weight, which includes a whole new level of delicious and nutritious options on the list, as your calorie and macro allowance increases one last time. Your calorie intake should be between 1,500 to 2,300 per day, consisting of more protein, carbohydrates, and fat, depending on your level of exercise, gender, height, and personal goals. In this phase, healthy eating habits along with next-level, personal care become second nature, and sustaining your new, healthy body weight evolves into a higher lifestyle.

MacroWise makes it easy to maintain the lifestyle by posting this expansive list of curated foods, beverages, and other categories on our website for free. Each item on the list is marked by *MacroWise Phase* – "Thin", "Lean", and "Healthy", so it's simple to choose the right foods for the phase you're in. All items have been carefully chosen based on their ingredients, number of calories, and nutritional value. Eating the selected foods for the phase you're in helps you stay within your macro range and lose weight as you transition through the 3 phases of MacroWise. You don't have to obsess over macronutrient ratios or understand the science behind nutrition because it's all done for you. By following the plan, you will know exactly what to eat and when to eat it. Everything you need to be thin, lean, and healthy is provided for you in this book and on our website. MacroWise.com is your gateway to locate and purchase the highest quality, low-sugar, macro-friendly foods from multiple online stores and local grocery stores. By following this replacement method of fueling up with foods from the list 6X a day every 2 ½ hours, your appetite will be satisfied, and you will lose weight permanently.

Most people never satisfy their appetite because they don't plan their food throughout the day, which leads to unhealthy snacking, delayed meals, and overeating. Snacking on sugary foods throughout the day delays eating nutritious, essential meals the body requires to function optimally. This lack of consistent nutrition deprives the body of vital protein, which causes muscles to deteriorate and leads to overeating the wrong foods at mealtime. The fact is, most people don't know what or when to eat, which is why we have an overweight society. Combining this lack of knowledge with the explosion of cheap, tasty junk food everywhere is the main reason for an overfed and undernourished, obese society. By knowing what and when to eat, combined with the determination to be thin, you can help yourself break free from being a mental and physical slave to food.

To be emotionally healthy, we need to believe that if we take action X, it can influence result Y. *Learned helplessness*, a term coined by psychologist Martin Seligman, occurs when a person feels that since they are not in control, they might as well give up. Seligman maintains that people have a perception of helplessness when they believe that their actions will not be able to influence their outcomes.

As an analogy, full-grown circus elephants are kept tethered with small ropes looped around one leg. They don't try to break free because they have been tethered in this way since they were young and weak. After trying repeatedly to break free without success, they give up. As adult elephants, they could easily tear the whole circus tent down and move about at will, but they have learned to be helpless, so they don't even try.

As a comparison, over the years we accepted excessive weight gain as a normal way of life. We assumed that growing in age meant growing in body weight and size. So, we allowed ourselves to be lulled into an unhealthy lifestyle that made us fat and tired. Many of us wanted to change our lives but didn't know how so we gave up. As time passed, new diets emerged but we didn't think they would work for us, so we stopped trying. We didn't believe there was an easy way out, so we learned to be helpless and gained a lot of weight in the process.

The bottom line is once you find a simple way to break free from being a slave to food then why not do it now? That's the premise behind *The Secret to Being Thin*. MacroWise gives you knowledge of what and when to eat, along with support to help you change. Our extensive list of tasty, healthy, macro-friendly foods and drinks is designed to melt your fat off if you stay committed to it. You don't have to exercise because the foods on the list have the right number of calories and macronutrients you need to burn fat. By sticking to the list and following the MacroWise rules, you will like everything you eat and lose weight consistently.

Contrary to the popular Nike slogan: "Just do it", when it comes to losing weight permanently, you shouldn't just do it. You must first "get a good plan...and then do it." It needs to be in that order. Otherwise, you will waste a lot of precious time on bad plans that cause you to give up forever. It's good to know there is a better way to enjoy food, stay satisfied, and be thin. You will see real results within 90 days of adopting the MacroWise lifestyle. Everything you need to make it happen for yourself is right here in this book and on our website. Simply trust the science, commit to the lifestyle, and watch the weight disappear fast and easily!

CHAPTER THREE

Changing Your Perception of What Food Means to You

I had 3 surgeries in 1 year and spent the next 15 years hooked on painkillers, anti-anxiety drugs, and sleeping pills. I spent most of those years trying to get off addictive, prescription drugs with no success. Over time, my daily dose increased along with my tolerance, and I became a drug addict. The physical pain from my surgeries went away, but if I didn't keep taking the pills every day, I would feel sick, anxious, and hungry for drugs. I knew that having the will to change was not enough on its own. A person needs a good plan that works. Otherwise, breaking free from any addiction becomes a vicious cycle of relapse and recovery. The moment I found a good plan to get off drugs, I quickly got clean and never relapsed again.

Food and sugar addictions are very similar to drug addiction. Just like popping pills whenever you feel like it, eating whatever you want whenever you feel like it can turn a person into a food addict. Since refined sugar is just as addictive as drugs like cocaine and heroin, the brain and body are vulnerable to sugar addiction and withdrawal. Once addicted, if you don't constantly consume your high-sugar foods, you feel sick, anxious, and hungry. Much like addictive drugs, sugar hijacks your brain by releasing huge surges of a neurotransmitter called dopamine. This hormone makes you feel good and causes you to want more. Once sugar leaves the body and dopamine levels drop, you instantly crave foods that contain sugar so you can feel good again. As a result, your brain tricks you into thinking you're hungry, so you end up eating more junk food which makes you fat and addicted. Simply put, consuming sugar triggers you to overeat and gain weight.

We all know that food is a necessary part of life and vital for survival. However, over the years, we've been programmed by mass media and society to believe that it's ok to eat whatever we want whenever we feel like it. I grew up having easy access to all the junk food I ever wanted. Snacking all day until late at night, was a normal way of life for me. Over time, my perception of what food meant to me became corrupted, which is how I formed bad eating habits and got fat. Just like getting off drugs, I couldn't break out of this unhealthy lifestyle until I admitted I had a problem and found a good plan for change.

I'm 6'5" and weighed 265 pounds the day my sister introduced me to a macro-diet she was promoting as a coach. The diet allowed a total intake of 800 to 1,000 calories per day and came with a strong emphasis on eating low-sugar, low-fat, and moderate carbs until you reached your goal weight. Since I'm very tall and had a lot of muscle from years of weightlifting when I was younger, I naturally assumed that I needed far more food than what her diet allowed. I had no clue that eating low-sugar, low-calorie, macro-friendly snacks, containing 10 grams of protein every 2 ½ hours would satisfy the needs of my big body. And discovering tasty, fast, easy-to-make meals, would make losing weight a real pleasure. It took a few days to detox from sugar before I realized that I was never hungry while following the rules of the diet. If I felt hungry after eating a protein snack, I would tell myself to "wait for it" because I knew that my body had what it needed, and the hunger pangs would go away in a few minutes. After making some simple adjustments to the way I ate, I proceeded to lose 2 ½ pounds every week until all the weight came off.

My perception of what food means to me soon changed from emotional eating to intellectual feeding. I evolved from binging on comfort food whenever I felt like it, to enjoying tasty, required sustenance on a well-timed schedule. I understood that if I consumed sugar, skipped fuelings, or delayed meals, I would end up eating the wrong foods at the wrong time, which would cause me to gain fat, lose muscle, and feel sluggish. I soon realized that by fueling up with the right number of calories and macros

6 times a day every 2 ½ hours, my body received exactly what it needed to burn fat, promote muscle growth, and sustain an active lifestyle. Consistently following this simple eating rule was the answer to speeding up my metabolism, losing weight, and changing my perception of what food means to me. Having a long list of tasty, low-sugar, low-calorie options, empowered me to remain consistent and reach my goal weight fast.

After reaching my goal body weight within 6 months, I began to enjoy some of my favorite foods again. However, I knew when to eat them and how to make healthy choices. To this present day, I continue to use the app on my phone to remind me to eat 6 times a day every 2 ½ hours. And I naturally practice healthy eating habits as a way of life whether at home or on the go. Everything I eat tastes good, satisfies my hunger, and is designed to maintain my goal weight. There is nothing I miss about my old, fat lifestyle.

Much like my experience with getting off drugs, eating clean and losing weight consistently for 6 months did not mean that I was cured of my old ways. Relapse is a normal part of recovery and always lurking around the corner. It usually occurs when you're experiencing unpleasant emotions from the negative side of life, such as sadness, anger, and fear. Maybe you're unhappy with the way your body looks, or you've had a bad day at work, are having financial issues, or are fighting with family. Binge eating can also occur when you're experiencing pleasant emotions from the positive side of life such as joy, love, and peace. Maybe you're happy with the way your body looks, had a good day at work, received a financial windfall, or reconciled with your family. You don't need one specific reason to relapse either. A binge can occur from a series of events that converge into one breaking point in time, which can then turn into a full-blown relapse.

I recall planning my first major eating binge about 6 months after reaching my goal weight of 215 pounds. I was on the phone getting ready to order all my old, favorite foods from Uber Eats. I remember being very excited about the process, kind of like the way I used to feel when procuring drugs. It was like my inner animal was taking over and I wanted to go along for the ride. It was easy to justify a binge after eating clean for a year. Plus, at the time I was dealing with a lot of stress from work, had financial issues, and was fighting with my family. The pressure was mounting, and I was looking for some relief. Ironically, the day I planned my binge with Uber Eats was a positive day because most of my problems cleared up. So, I'm not sure what specifically triggered me on that day since I was feeling fine.

Maybe I was trying to use junk food as a way of getting pleasure to make up for my prior pain. Maybe I was more susceptible to a binge on that day because I was running low on sleep. Maybe I was able to justify a dirty binge since, unlike drug addiction, I could afford to take a "day off" because I knew I had the discipline to return the next day. Or perhaps I was just bored and wanted to have a little fun.

Regardless of any reason, I managed to stop myself from placing the order by asking myself if I wanted to go down this path. I reasoned with myself by considering whether it was wise to give in at this point. Where was this binge going to lead me? What benefit do I gain from it? What will this choice cost me? What does food mean to me? What is the real purpose of food? Was I trying to use food like a drug to feel good? Unlike drug addiction, we can take a moment to pause, breathe, and consider our food options, before we act. As healthy human beings, we can choose to guide our emotions intelligently and make better decisions. Just because we want to do something that makes us feel good, that doesn't mean we have to do it.

I also considered the fact that my kitchen was stocked with macro-wise ingredients for making anything I could order through Uber Eats. I had low-carb pita bread, marinara sauce, vegan pepperoni, and shredded cheese in the fridge if I wanted pizza. I could take some low-carb buns and lean ground beef out of the freezer, add cheese and condiments from the refrigerator, and enjoy a good cheeseburger. And if I wanted to order out because I didn't feel like cooking, there were plenty of tasty, clean options to choose from. I didn't have to order the wrong foods, nor did I have to overeat. Regardless of any situation life throws at you, whether good or bad, it's important to know you always have choices. You don't have to revert to your old ways, since there are plenty of macro-wise options all around you. And even though there's nothing wrong with rewarding yourself from time-to-time, you need to remember it's a slippery slope, and you should watch yourself objectively to avoid falling.

"Being thin feels better than food tastes"...someone told me that a long time ago and it stuck with me because it's very true. However, you don't have to give up eating tasty food to be thin. You can have your cake and eat it too, so long as the cake is from the MacroWise list. MacroWise is your proven plan to lose weight, get in shape, and live healthily. The main thing required from you is for you to decide to change and follow the plan. As you progress through the MacroWise lifestyle, your perception of what food means to you will change for the better and you will never look back!

CHAPTER FOUR

Trauma, Stress & Food Addiction

The underlying cause behind most addictions is trauma. The link between trauma and addiction has many painful origins, which can be difficult to identify and heal. Trauma can be the result of child abuse, sexual abuse, neglect, abandonment, the death of a loved one, domestic violence, poverty, divorce, bullying, a physical accident, and many more. Any one of these traumatic events can leave lasting mental damage known as PTSD, which often develops into various addictions. In addition to a major trauma, experiencing a high frequency of smaller, stressful events over time can create an acute trauma that also fuels addiction. It's a simple fact that life hurts from time to time. Mental and physical pain creates a desire to escape into various forms of pleasure. The fastest way to avoid feeling bad is by doing something easy that makes you feel good. Repeating this pattern of escapism over time turns a person into an addict. Regardless of the underlying cause of your addiction, it's imperative to realize that you are not your trauma. The connection between trauma and addiction is a complicated issue that can't be resolved here in a few paragraphs. However, a person needs to know that once they admit to having a problem and make the decision to change, breaking any addiction is possible.

In the previous chapter, I mentioned that I had 3 surgeries in 1 year and spent the next 15 years hooked on drugs and junk food. I spent most of those years trying to break free from my addictions with little to no success. The reason I didn't explain the various factors that led to my addictions was that we all have pain and stress in our lives. It's up to each of us to identify the cause of our pain, process the emotions, and let go, so we can finally move on with our lives.

So, after acknowledging that I was stuck in a rut and powerless against my addictions, I decided to move 2,700 miles away to achieve a mental, physical, and emotional reset. Even though I had little money at the time, I didn't put any conditions on my decision to move. I knew there was never going to be a perfect time and life was quickly passing by, so I mustered up the courage and moved from Florida to California. I made sure to relocate to a place where I wasn't surrounded by negativity. I committed to getting back to doing some of the favorite pastimes I once enjoyed before drug addiction took over my life.

I began my self-healing journey by focusing on breaking my toughest addiction, which was a variety of mind-altering, prescription drugs. I knew that if I overcame my greatest challenge, I could conquer anything. I researched all the ways to get off prescription drugs and found a natural replacement method that felt right to me. I then began the process of detoxing and rehabbing from opioids, which was my drug of choice. After spending years trying to get clean, it only took 30 days to taper me off painkillers. What followed was months of rehabilitation. My recovery included practicing mental coping skills and establishing physical replacement pleasures that made sobriety a breeze. Within a few months of working on my recovery, I transformed old, toxic patterns into new, healthy habits. Once the opioids were out of my system, I started to see value in myself and the world around me. My perception of reality was getting lighter and brighter, and I embraced the positive change.

Even though I suffered from mental and physical pain throughout my drug recovery, I started doing some light exercises. I walked outside every night and explored the new sights and sounds around me. I remember the first night I began, I could barely walk half a mile with my mind and body kicking and screaming the whole way. I chose to ignore the negative chatter in my head, and instead increased the amount of distance I walked each night. Half a mile of walking soon turned into several miles, which eventually led to resistance training. Getting off drugs motivated me to rehabilitate my body, after years of abusing and neglecting it.

A couple of months into my recovery from opioid addiction, I started the same process of detoxing and rehabbing from anti-anxiety medication, referred to as benzodiazepines. It turns out that detoxing from this type of prescription drug is far more difficult than opioids because it takes a lot longer to leave the body. Regardless, I knew I could do it after my success with getting off painkillers. So, I proceeded to taper off benzodiazepines in just 30 days, by using the same natural replacement method and applying the same coping skills. This simple method enabled me to ease my painful withdrawal symptoms and nullify my cravings while getting off each drug. I systematically eliminated one substance at a time, until I was clean and free from all drugs.

The last remaining addiction from my old, toxic lifestyle was staring me in the face every time I got out of the shower and looked in the mirror. I knew it was time to get off junk food and lose body fat. I searched and found a natural replacement method like the one I used for getting off drugs and applied it to lose 2 ½ pounds every week until I reached my goal body weight. Food is a necessary part of life, which is why many claim it's one of the hardest addictions to overcome. We must eat to live, but that doesn't mean we should live to eat. We're programmed by mass media and society to believe that it's normal to eat whatever we want whenever we feel like it. Unfortunately, permissible pleasures often lead to overindulgence and addiction. This slippery slope coupled with pain from the past, helps to explain why so many people are grossly overweight even though it's unhealthy and unattractive.

People can make the argument that trauma and stress in their lives have nothing to do with their addiction, which may be true for some. I've heard plenty of drug addicts say they only use drugs because they like the way it makes them feel, but that's not the whole truth. Obese people love the way food makes them feel which is their excuse for overeating and being fat, but that's not the whole truth either. For years, I abused food to get temporary relief from feeling bad. Anytime I wanted to escape from feeling bored, sad, or lonely, I turned to the junk-food drawer. Sugar was an easy drug for me to get as a kid because junk food was permissible in my house, and I had a free, unlimited supply. I assumed that my lifestyle was normal and had little interest in changing.

Multiple experiments show that individuals who are exposed to unpleasant conditions they cannot control will become withdrawn. In one such experiment, subjects were exposed to extremely high levels of noise. By pushing a button, one group could stop the noise while the other could not stop the noise. A short while later when both groups were brought together, individuals from the group who could do nothing about the noise – and were helpless – when asked to participate in a sports game, showed little interest or motivation to win (Hiroto, D.: Learned helplessness, In: *Journal of Experimental Psychology*, 1974).

Overcoming trauma, stress, and food addiction is attainable when you have the desire, knowledge, and determination to change. You can spend a lifetime going in the wrong direction, and then turn it all around on any given day. It's critical to know that you are not your past, and it's never too late to change. You can achieve a new "I.D." by "identifying and dissolving" old, bad patterns in your life, and replacing them with new, good habits. The power to win is yours once you decide to change and start applying the simple principles you gain from this book. The knowledge and support you receive here will motivate you to create a new life by breaking the painful cycle of trauma, stress, and food addiction.

You can achieve lasting change by adopting the MacroWise lifestyle. If you want real, professional help to get started and don't want to waste any more time, we recommend using our MacroWise coaching service to show you the way. We have daily instructional videos, as well as live phone coaches to guide you through the weight-loss process and keep you motivated. Working with a coach helped me and many others just like you to lose weight, get in shape, and live healthy. Regardless of your reasons for being overweight, the secret to being thin is yours once you get MacroWise!

CHAPTER FIVE

Sugar Is the Enemy!

The greatest enemy a person can encounter is an invisible terrorist because there's no way to identify it and protect yourself from an attack. When it comes down to a person who wants to lose weight, sugar is that invisible terrorist because it's mixed into so many of the foods we eat every day. Unless you have a trained eye, it's very difficult to identify this hidden enemy and protect yourself from getting hurt.

Most overweight people think they can lose weight by making a few, clever tweaks to the way they eat, like a sandwich with wheat bread instead of white, a salad with a quarter cup of ranch dressing instead of a half cup, a fruit smoothie instead of a big gulp soda, or a side of brown rice instead of French fries. Unfortunately, this mentality of eating less junk to lose weight only keeps a person stuck in an ignorant, perpetual cycle of sugar dependency, withdrawal, and food addiction.

I'm not a doctor, scientist, or registered dietician, but I've gained real experience through overcoming drug addiction. And I guarantee you that sugar is a highly addictive, dangerous drug that's responsible for a worldwide epidemic of sick, fat people. The lasting health damage caused by using this drug over time is easy for anyone to research and verify. There are many popular documentaries, books, and medical studies found online that illustrate this fact far better than I can here. The main point you need to know is that an overweight person trying to lose weight can't eat sugary foods and expect to be thin. Just like a recovering cocaine addict can't use their drug and expect to maintain their sobriety. In both cases, the addict's occasional use of drugs fuels a vicious cycle of relapse and addiction.

Overeating and gaining weight are typically the result of sugar addiction and withdrawal. Since sugar is mixed into most foods like an invisible terrorist, you're likely to overeat and gain weight because sugar makes you think you're hungry. As the "sugar drug" leaves the body, your nervous system sends messages to the brain which makes you want to eat foods that contain sugar. This is no different than a cocaine addict coming off their drug and needing to do more drugs to feel normal again. The reality is, you don't need to eat any more food. You just need to know that you're in sugar withdrawal and should refrain from giving in by feeding your brain and body more. Once you stop sugar and get MacroWise, you will not crave junk food anymore. Your brain will no longer trick you into thinking you're hungry since MacroWise replaces sugar with sweet, non-addictive, wholesome ingredients.

As a result of significantly reducing sugar intake and increasing protein intake, your desire to snack on junk food throughout the day will go away. The fake hunger pangs will disappear because your brain and body will be calm and satisfied. You need to remember that the lifestyle of eating whatever you want whenever you feel like it, is responsible for your weight gain. The days of eating whatever and whenever will finally stop along with your cravings after you start MacroWise. This program helps you make simple tweaks to your lifestyle that create healthy eating habits and produce lasting change.

The biggest challenge to overcome when starting a low-sugar diet is the process of detoxing your brain and body from sugar. The withdrawal symptoms you will experience are similar to detoxing from addictive drugs, but nowhere near as bad. Common symptoms of sugar withdrawal include cravings and fatigue, but in some cases, people experience irritability, depressed mood, and other unwanted symptoms. For people on very low-sugar diets such as the ketogenic diet, sugar withdrawal can feel so severe and unpleasant that it is referred to as the "keto flu." The nature and severity of these symptoms vary from one person to the next. They usually last for a few days but can persist for up to a few weeks. Some additional symptoms you may experience when cutting sugar from your diet are anxiety, nausea, changes in sleep patterns, difficulty concentrating, dizziness, and lightheadedness. Plus, naturally, there's going to be cravings for sweets and carbohydrates like cookies, chips, pasta, sodas, and more.

These symptoms can be unpleasant, and cravings can lead to binge-eating behaviors. While experiencing a period of sugar withdrawal, people often give in to cravings and end up consuming a bunch of junk food. Binge-eating is part of the vicious cycle of sugar addiction and withdrawal. After a binge, people often feel guilty, depressed, and angry. To make themselves feel better, they eat more foods that contain sugar to get the endorphins and dopamine flowing again. Dopamine makes you feel good while eating junk, but that doesn't last long.

Sugar withdrawal doesn't require long-term treatment because it passes relatively quickly. The main problem for most people on restrictive diets, such as keto, is sustaining a low-sugar lifestyle, which is one of the reasons why many drop out. Very few people know which foods to buy to avoid sugar. Much like an invisible terrorist, sugar is a tricky enemy to identify. It's in many of the healthy foods we eat, including fruit, bread, and dairy products. The key to changing bad eating habits is to find a good plan for replacing sugar that you can live with.

One of the main reasons why MacroWise works is because our snacks contain low-sugar, low-calorie, quality ingredients, and are portion-controlled with the right number of macros. MacroWise offers a vast variety of delicious foods that use healthy, all-natural sweeteners, like monk fruit, organic dark chocolate, cacao butter, tapioca fiber, cane sugar, yacon syrup, chocolate liquor, cocoa, cinnamon, vanilla extract, almond butter, and more. These ingredients are used in making some of the world's tastiest foods and provide a natural replacement for sugar. In addition, MacroWise snacks contain protein that comes from quality, natural sources, like hemp, peas, lentils, beans, rice, seeds, nuts, collagen, tofu, whey, milk, eggs, fish, chicken, and meat. The combination of tasty, healthy foods that are low in calories and high in clean protein, ensures you stay satisfied and lose weight the right way.

The purpose of MacroWise is to lose weight through eating clean, which is why you should avoid consuming low-calorie, sugar-free drinks that contain toxic, artificial ingredients. Studies have shown that artificial sweeteners may cause a range of health problems, such as headaches, diabetes, heart disease, cancer, and obesity. Many people consume sugar-free, carbonated beverages because they provide fewer calories than sugar-sweetened alternatives. However, the artificial sweeteners in these drinks may lead to weight gain. According to an article published in the "Yale Journal of Biology and Medicine" in June 2010, consuming natural sweeteners activates food reward pathways in your brain, but artificial sweeteners don't fully activate these pathways. This can leave you feeling unsatisfied and lead to an increased appetite, even if you've already eaten enough calories for the day. The intensely sweet flavor of artificial sweeteners may also trigger cravings for sugary food and lead to excess calorie intake. Regardless of what the billion-dollar advertising campaigns say about enjoying their low-calorie, sugar-free junk, do not buy into the hype by thinking it will help you lose weight.

There are no shortcuts in life, but soon after you adopt the MacroWise lifestyle, you will realize there is a better way to enjoy food and be thin at the same time. You will no longer stand in front of your open refrigerator at night contemplating bad choices because you will know exactly what to eat and when to eat it. Our entire list of macro-friendly foods tastes great and provides maximum nutrition, without the high calories or sugar. You will not miss any of your favorite foods from the past because macro-wise foods satisfy. The secret to being thin is here for you once you decide to stop using sugar and get MacroWise.

We understand that everyone is different, and some people require special attention because of various mental, physical, or religious reasons. So, we also have many organic, vegan, gluten-free, and kosher options to choose from on our list of curated foods. And, if you're looking for help beyond our daily coaching videos and texting service, we also offer next-level support with our highly trained, one-on-one phone coaches. They can address all your special needs and dietary restrictions to create a custom food plan that works best for you. It's good to know that MacroWise offers professional support to guide you through one of the toughest, personal struggles facing our generation today.

CHAPTER SIX

A Manual for Feeding the Human Body

The reason why a person fails to learn and practice various fundamental truths in life is usually the result of having bad teachers and role models. It does not matter whether you chose the person as your teacher or if the person was chosen for you because the outcome is often the same. If the teacher you chose is skilled in teaching but unaware the information they are spreading is false, you will believe the lie and practice it. Likewise, if the teacher that was chosen for you has true information to share but doesn't effectively communicate it, you will also fail to learn and practice the truth. We could all be good students, teachers, and role models if a true manual for higher living was given to us by a good teacher.

One of the reasons why so many people are overweight is because we were never given a proper manual for feeding the human body by a good teacher. Growing up in the public school system in the 80's, taught me there are 4 basic food groups a person should stick to for healthy eating: fruits & vegetables, grains, dairy, and meat. Subsequently, our school's cafeteria served macaroni & cheese, pizza, corndogs, steak & cheese subs, French fries, fruit cocktail, and chocolate milk for lunch. As a result, my perception of an ideal, healthy meal as a kid was a meat & vegetable pizza with a tall glass of fruit punch. It contained all 4 food groups and was congruent with what I learned from my food teachers. The people chosen to be my teachers fed me bad information, which caused me to be ignorant and get fat. But, since junk food tastes so good, I didn't bother looking for a better teacher!

In addition to food, there are many examples of how bad teachers and role models have led us astray in life. The healthcare system in America programs us from birth to accept prescription drugs as a true solution for most health problems. Big Pharma accounts for 75% of all paid television advertising in the U.S., which is why so many people are okay with using RX drugs. Being exposed to such a high frequency of TV ads has a profound effect on a person's belief system and perception of reality. It's easy to see how someone can normalize the regular use of prescription drugs, as health issues surface throughout one's life. When I had 3 surgeries in 1 year, my doctors wrote me countless prescriptions for opioids, benzodiazepines, and sleeping pills. After a few months of popping happy pills every day, I became a drug addict. I listened to my esteemed teachers because I assumed they knew what was best. Plus, the drugs made me feel good, so I didn't bother looking for a better teacher!

The tobacco industry was spending a fortune on television advertising to promote the many "benefits" of smoking cigarettes until they were banned from TV in 1971. Some of these TV commercials used doctors dressed in white lab coats to endorse smoking as a healthy pastime. Other TV ads showed famous actors looking good, being cool, and loving life while enjoying a cigarette. The power of TV or "Tel-Lie-Vision" was, is, and always will be, used by nefarious corporations to seduce you into buying their junk. People are more likely to purchase a product without questioning its integrity when being promoted by someone they look up to as a role model. Albert Einstein was once quoted as saying, "I believe that pipe smoking contributes to a somewhat calm and objective judgment in all human affairs." Sadly, cigarette smoking is estimated to cause 480,000 deaths in the U.S. annually. Cigarette smoking remains the leading cause of preventable disease, disability, and death in the United States. Whether it's smoking cigarettes, drinking alcohol, taking prescription drugs, or eating junk food, the money-hungry role models you choose, along with the "black screen", play a major role in harming the masses.

I recall going to sleepaway camp as a boy for the first time and experiencing a community bathroom. I met some kid in the bathroom who started talking to me while I was brushing my teeth. He told me that his dad was a dentist and proceeded to teach me the right way to brush my teeth. I knew his information was true because my dentist already told me the same things, except the kid added something new. His method included swallowing the remaining toothpaste in his mouth at the end of the session. His flavor of choice was bubble gum, and he clearly enjoyed eating it. He tried to convince me to do the same by telling me it freshens your breath and tastes great. I later learned that most toothpaste contains fluoride, which is a very poisonous mineral. If you swallow any amount, you're supposed to call poison control and go to the hospital's emergency room immediately. Medical studies have shown that fluoride causes many types of horrible diseases and permanently lowers a person's IQ. Someone must have taught that boy it was okay to swallow toothpaste, and then he chose to pass it on to others, which is how the cycle of ignorance continues. Fortunately for me, I didn't listen to that kid and swallow toothpaste, but sadly many do. Regardless, it's easy to see how something so innocent as brushing your teeth every day can be corrupted and eventually compromise your health if left unchecked.

There is an overwhelming amount of misinformation and disinformation constantly being broadcasted all around us. Most of that bad information is being channeled to us by greedy corporations and ignorant role models. It's your job to question everything you see, hear, and read, so you can discern between what you thought was true and the truth. You can start by inspecting your personal care routine and throwing out any products that contain harmful, toxic ingredients. Assess your healthcare system to make sure your doctors have not exposed you to unnecessary medical treatments that may be detrimental to your health. And of course, you need to investigate everything you eat and drink to determine if your food choices are being influenced by bad role models and the black screen.

You must learn to be a critical thinker who questions all the information you've accepted as truth over the years. For example, is the Earth a spinning ball of water flying through space or a stationary, flat plane? Does gravity exist or does matter simply weigh more than air? Is the moon a floating, physical rock that you can land on or a spiritual luminary? Did humans evolve from apes or are we spiritual beings living in a physical body designed by a higher power? Regardless of how wacky these questions may sound, we are living in a world of lies and now is the time to wake up, stand up, and make some wise adjustments to our lives.

Throughout the world, there's a pandemic of addiction taking place. People are hooked on many forms of junk, such as sugar, vapor, cigarettes, alcohol, drugs, gambling, pornography, and technology. These days, more and more people are staying indoors, hooked to their black screens, and living a sedentary lifestyle. It's understandable why so many people are lonely, depressed, and overweight. Your role models inside the black screen keep you glued to your electronics and are not going to show you how to break free from screen addiction. Nor is your friendly healthcare provider likely to prescribe natural remedies for your medical ailments outside of the goliath, healthcare system. And the big food and beverage companies pushing their junk on every street corner are not going to recommend healthy options for you to eat and drink outside of their domain either.

You spent many years listening to bad teachers, celebrity influencers, seductive advertising campaigns, and your inner animal's insatiable appetite for pleasure. Once you realize that many of your teachers have been leading you down the wrong path, it's your responsibility to seek out good teachers and take the right path. MacroWise provides you with the knowledge and support to walk the true path by conditioning in new, healthy eating habits that you own for life. Fueling your body with the right foods at the right time is essential for losing fat and maintaining a healthy body. Conversely, failure to consistently provide your body with clean fuel on a well-timed schedule causes it to age and deteriorate. Medical studies have linked bad eating habits and obesity to premature aging and disease. Fortunately, a person's youthful appearance and vitality quickly return when they lose weight by eating wisely.

People often take extreme paths when trying to lose weight fast. Some people starve themselves, which harms the brain and body over time. Most turn to unsustainable fad diets, so they relapse and end up gaining even more weight. All extremes are unwise, which is why someone serious about losing weight permanently should take the middle path. This book is your manual for taking the wise, middle path to losing weight and maintaining your goal weight. The book teaches you that eating the foods from the list 6X a day every 2 ½ hours and staying within your calorie and macro range are the secrets to being thin.

People need a good food teacher with true information and no agenda other than helping them succeed in achieving their ideal body. MacroWise makes it possible for all of us to be good students, teachers, and role models by giving you a manual for feeding the human body.

CHAPTER SEVEN

The Art of Micro-Eating

In previous chapters, I explained how I was addicted to prescription drugs for 15 years. The moment I found a good plan for getting off drugs, I got serious about getting sober and took decisive action. Within a few months, I was clean from 3 different types of highly addictive, prescription drugs. Throughout that time, I experienced minimal pain and cravings, which are common withdrawal symptoms that lead to relapse. I was able to achieve those amazing results through the art of microdosing with natural medicine. The medicine I used to detox was a combination of high-milligram CBD and low-milligram THC. There are many medicinal benefits found in CBD, but it requires a little bit of THC to activate the healing power within. This combination of ingesting large amounts of CBD oil, along with very small amounts of THC oil, provided me with the mental and physical relief I needed to make it through detox and stay clean. This natural replacement method was my secret for replacing bad with good and making lasting changes.

Before starting my drug detox, I experimented with different dosages of cannabis oil to determine which amount worked best for me. I surmised the accurate dose to ingest was 250mg of CBD oil plus 2.5mg of THC oil, 6X a day every 2 ½ hours. If I took too much THC, I would get too high and want to use my old drugs again. If I didn't take enough THC, the physical pain and cravings from withdrawal would persist, which would also cause me to want to use drugs again. I started my drug detox once I figured out the precise microdose of THC needed to feel normal throughout detox. I spent 30 days tapering off each prescription drug, while I simultaneously micro-dosed THC oil to ease the withdrawal symptoms. The art of microdosing a natural substance to detox from an addictive drug demonstrates the power of taking the non-extreme, middle path to making lasting change.

I know plenty of people who tried using cannabis medicinally but were scared off by the negative side effects, like paranoia, anxiety, and the munchies. I've heard many stories of people who felt like they were going to have a heart attack or go crazy after eating a high-milligram THC gummy. Very few people know the precise dose needed to feel the way they want, so they eat too much THC and have a bad reaction as a result. Cannabis can be used as a healthy alternative to alcohol and prescription drugs for alleviating various mental, physical, emotional, and spiritual issues, such as trauma, pain, stress, and depression. Once you teach someone that con-suming less medicine portioned out over time provides more benefits, they will likely value the art of microdosing. This art requires some knowledge and discipline. However, the reward for practicing it is very great.

Many good examples demonstrate microdosing as an effective solu-tion for your well-being. One of those examples can be found in hydrating. Drinking water every day is essential for staying hydrated. The National Academy of Medicine recommends that adult women and men drink 90 and 125 ounces of water a day. (For context, one gallon is 128 fluid ounc-es.) But pounding large amounts of water morning, noon, and night, may not be the best or most efficient way to meet the body's hydration require-ments. Research shows that sipping water or "micro-drinking" throughout the day provides better hydration than gulping a large amount in a short time. The popular idea that constant and heavy water consumption flushes the body of toxins or unwanted material is a half-truth. While urine does transport chemical byproducts and waste out of the body, drinking lots of water on an empty stomach doesn't improve this cleansing process.

"If you're drinking lots of water and then, within two hours, your urine output is high and your urine is clear, that means the water is not staying in well. In fact, clear urine is a sign of overhydration," according to the Cleveland Clinic. "Guzzling lots of water is not the best way to stay hydrated. In some rare cases, excessive water consumption can even be harmful. There are better ways to keep the body and brain hydrated than to pound water all day long. Sipping water a little bit at a time prevents the kidneys from being overloaded and helps the body retain more H20." – *David Nieman, a professor of public health at Appalachian State University and director of the Human Performance Lab at the North Carolina Research Campus.* Nieman says - "the take-home message isn't that people should drink less water, nor that they should swap out water for other beverages. But for those hoping to stay optimally hydrated, a slow-and-steady approach to water consumption and coupling water with little food is a more effective method than knocking back full glasses of H20 between meals." Drinking water is a necessary part of life, but much like food and drugs, you can drown in it too.

Another good example that demonstrates the art of microdosing and how to apply it in our everyday lives is something we all naturally learn as children. Most kids have limited finances and rely on a small allowance to buy things. As a result, they're forced to spend within a modest budget. Knowing how to manage that budget early on serves as valuable training for the future. "Micro-budgeting" is the process of applying spending limits to programs and decisions. Instead of being foolish by making impulsive, emotional decisions, a person can choose to be wise by making cautious, emotionally intelligent decisions congruent with their higher goals. The art of micro-budgeting requires some calculating and discipline. However, the benefits of practicing it run deep.

As a kid, one of my favorite weekend pastimes was going to the mall with a friend. I would get dropped off around noon and get picked up at 8 pm with a budget of $20. We had an 8-hour routine that included the arcade, movie theater, food court, and store hopping. My goal was to have as much fun as possible during that time with a $20 budget. The arcade was my favorite spot in the mall, and I loved playing video games. They had good games that cost 25 cents each and amazing games that cost a buck. I could have easily blown my $20 budget within the first 3 hours if I wasn't careful. Instead, I allocated $4 over the next 2 hours before going to the movie theater. A movie ticket back then was $5. A soda and snack added another $3, which bought me 2 more hours of pleasure for $8. We would usually burn an hour before the movie started by walking around the mall and visiting our favorite stores. After the movie was over, we hit the food court. The cafeteria was one of my favorite places. I loved the variety of fast, delicious foods and bright, neon signs. There were many options to choose from, but I was mindful of my budget and ordered accordingly. $6 for dinner and another hour passes followed by 1 more hour of store hopping. My last $2 bought me 1 final hour at the arcade before I was picked up at 8 pm. If I had blown my budget in one shot, I would have spent most of the day bored and hungry. Instead, I spread my money out evenly over 8 hours and enjoyed the whole day. Practicing the art of micro-budgeting as a kid prepared me to calculate and enforce healthy boundaries and goals as an adult.

In addition to, microdosing medicine, water, and money, there's another form of microdosing that provides a simple solution for your weight management needs. The method of self-regulating your daily food consumption is a careful balancing act we refer to as the art of "micro-eating." The MacroWise method of eating smaller portions of low-sugar, nutrient-dense foods spread out evenly throughout the day is the secret to being thin. The MacroWise lifestyle personifies the art of micro-eating by providing you with a list of nutritious foods that you eat 6 times a day, every 2 ½ hours. Sticking to the list and following the basic rules ensures you consume the right number of calories and macros needed to burn fat and maintain muscle mass. When you exceed your daily calorie allowance, your body falls out of fat-burning mode and stops losing weight. It takes 3 to 5 days of micro-eating to put your metabolism back into fat-burning mode and start losing weight again. People who are determined to lose weight understand the consequences of exceeding their daily allowance and the importance of counting calories to avoid postponing their goals.

Since MacroWise limits your daily calorie intake, you must make sure the calories you consume are rich in protein. There's a big difference between eating a 150-calorie snack with 2 grams of protein vs. a 150-calorie snack with 10 grams of protein. Your body needs to be fed ample, clean protein consistently. Otherwise, your muscles will deteriorate, and your hunger will grow, causing you to overeat and gain weight. If your daily calorie allowance is only 1,300, then you need to make sure those calories are nutrient-dense and spread them out evenly throughout your waking hours. Even though 1,300 calories a day sounds so little, when those calories are high in protein and low in sugar, you will not be hungry until it's time to eat. Most of the foods people eat today are low in protein and high in sugar, which is why so many people are overfed and undernourished. Consuming 1,300 "macro-wise calories" a day typically provides far more nutrition and health benefits than consuming 4,000 "regular calories" a day. As you progress through the 3 phases of MacroWise, your daily calorie limit will increase from 1,300 to 2,300 calories which allows you to eat more of the foods you enjoy every day.

I mastered the art of micro-eating within 3 months of starting my weight-loss journey. I went from eating whatever I wanted whenever I felt like it, to eating the right foods from a curated list 6 times a day, every 2 ½ hours. During my first 90 days on the diet, I consumed between 1,000 to 1,300 calories a day consisting of 5 MacroWise snacks plus 1 MacroWise meal and no exercise. I made sure to keep my snacks around 150 calories. Each contained about 10 grams of protein, 15 grams of carbs, and 10 grams of fat. After the first 90 days and until I reached my goal weight, I consumed between 1,300 to 1,700 calories a day consisting of 4 MacroWise snacks plus 2 MacroWise meals and light exercise. I kept my snacks around 200 calories. Each contained more protein, carbs, and fat. After reaching my goal weight and maintaining it for a while, I consumed between 1,500 to 2,300 calories a day. That consisted of 1 to 3 MacroWise snacks plus 2 to 3 MacroWise meals and moderate exercise. I kept my snacks around 250 calories. Each contained more protein, carbs, and fat. If at any point I started to gain weight, I would quickly tighten up my calorie and carb intake to restart fat-burning mode. Even after maintaining my initial goal weight for a year, I went back to eating 5 MacroWise snacks plus 1 MacroWise meal a day for a few months to lose more weight. It's common to raise the bar and set a new goal weight after reaching your first one.

The art of micro-eating is like a food allowance given to you each day. There is a set limit to how much you get, so be mindful to spend it wisely and make it count.

CHAPTER EIGHT

Installing Healthy Eating Habits

Throughout this book, I make comparisons between breaking bad eating habits and overcoming drug addiction. They both have a lot in common considering junk food brings instant gratification similar to drugs. Some studies have suggested that sugar is just as addictive as cocaine because of the dopamine release people enjoy. In my opinion, it's much harder to break an addiction to drugs than to change a bad eating habit. The most important distinction between the two is how choice, to an extent, is still possible with habit-forming behaviors, like eating junk. But, when it comes to drug addiction, people generally have a harder time making decisions because of their dependence on such an extreme substance. It's impossible to think clearly or be rational when drug addiction takes over. If you go without sugar for a while, you will be fine because you can always eat other foods, and no harm will come to you. However, a drug addiction requires you to constantly use your drug. Otherwise, you feel like you're going to die. Unlike sugar, there are no clear options. The truth is, installing healthy eating habits was a piece of cake compared to breaking my addiction to drugs.

Just like many popular diets today, there are many programs for getting off drugs. One of my earlier attempts to get off painkillers led me to an ibogaine detox clinic. Ibogaine is a very powerful, psychedelic herb used for rapidly detoxing the brain and body from opioids. It's a simple treatment that consists of swallowing some herbal pills while lying in bed for 8 hours. When the psychedelic trip ends, all withdrawal symptoms and cravings for opiates are gone. After my ibogaine detox ended, a therapist at the clinic explained that my brain and body were clean from drugs. However, I still had the mental habit to overcome. Taking a few magic pills helped me stay sober for a little while, but it wasn't going to change the way I think or act long-term. Regardless of how many failed attempts to stop using drugs, I refused to see myself as a drug addict because I believed I was better than that. I knew it was just a matter of time before I got clean and lived my best life. Sadly, I wasted some of the best years of my life before realizing that vision. Drug addiction is one of the most difficult problems to overcome, and it took many bad years before I found a good plan for doing so.

Since overcoming drug addiction is more difficult than breaking bad eating habits, I knew it would be easy to change the way I ate once I found a good plan. Much like ingesting high-milligram CBD and low-milligram THC, 6 times a day, every 2 ½ hours to relieve my pain and nullify my cravings for drugs. I learned that eating high-protein, low-sugar foods, 6 times a day, every 2 ½ hours would satisfy my hunger and crush my cravings for junk food. I knew my replacement plan was working because I was quickly losing weight each week. At that point, it was easy to install healthy eating habits and create lasting change. There wasn't a good reason not to change. Since I enjoyed everything I ate, I was never hungry, and my body fat was melting away. After a few weeks of repeating this new way of eating and seeing positive results, my brain accepted the change and went along with it until it became a habit.

Regardless of whether your goal is to get off drugs, lose weight, or even get rich, having a good plan will fuel your persistence to achieve it. Ray Crock, the founder of McDonald's Corporation was a struggling businessman who spent most of his adult life looking for a good business plan to get rich. For years, Ray tried selling all kinds of products door-to-door both residentially and commercially. He was a 52-year-old traveling salesman who sold milkshake machines to diners when he met the McDonald brothers at their fast-food restaurant in California. Since Ray spent so much time traveling cross-country, he was forced to eat at diners along the way. Throughout that time, he learned about the downside to eating at those diners and felt there had to be a better way to serve people food. Once he discovered the tasty, inexpensive, fast-food experience at McDonald's, he knew that he finally found a good plan to get rich. Once he had that plan, he was persistent and determined to succeed.

Ray Crock was quoted years ago explaining the secret to his success. He said, "How the heck does a 52-year-old, over-the-hill, milkshake machine salesman build a fast-food empire with 1,600 restaurants in 50 states, 5 foreign countries, with an annual revenue of $700 million?... One word, persistence. Nothing in the world can take the place of good old persistence. Talent won't. Nothing is more common than unsuccessful men with talent. Genius won't. Unrewarded genius is practically a cliché. Education won't. The world is full of educated fools. Persistence and determination alone are all-powerful." Today, the McDonald's corporation is the most successful fast-food restaurant in the world. It has over 40,000 locations worldwide, generates 23 billion dollars in annual sales, and feeds 1% of the world's population every day.

Unfortunately, corporations like McDonald's have played a major role in creating an epidemic of obesity and disease. In the United States, 42% of adults have obesity, which means more than 1 out of 3 people are over-weight. Plus, 1 out of 11 adults have severe obesity and suffer from an extreme case of food addiction. Worldwide, obesity is a common problem and a major health issue associated with numerous diseases, specifically an increased risk of certain types of cancer, coronary artery disease, type 2 diabetes, cardiovascular disease, and stroke as well as significant increases in mortality and economic costs. The estimated annual medical cost of obesity in the United States alone is around $200 billion. Medical costs for adults who are obese are about $2,000 higher per year than medical costs for people with healthy weight. So, even though eating fast food appears to be cheaper in the short term, the monetary costs associated with the deterioration of your physical health are far more expensive in the long term.

Much like Ray Crock was persistent about succeeding in business, you can do the same in your personal life by being persistent about losing weight. It's much easier to accomplish your goal when you have a good plan that works, especially when that plan involves improving your health and appearance as opposed to destroying it with junk like fast food. Knowing you have a good plan gives you the confidence and willpower to persist. Regardless of how good your plan is, starting something new in life is the hardest thing to do. But once you start your weight-loss journey with MacroWise, sticking to it quickly becomes a habit. You follow the process one day at a time and the positive results soon reveal themselves. The first day turns into weeks and then months. Eventually, healthy eating habits become second nature. You won't deviate from the plan because nothing is worth it once you've discovered the power of MacroWise. By sticking to the plan, you naturally install healthy eating habits that empower you to reach your goal weight and maintain it for life.

I'm determined to maintain my goal weight forever, which is why I strictly enforce it. This number is non-negotiable, which means the amount I weigh is almost always the same. I reached a point in my life where I refused to let myself weigh any more. I've maintained this number for a while and do not allow it to increase. I still enjoy all my favorite foods, so long as the ingredients are from the MacroWise list. Whether it's tacos, fajitas, cheeseburgers, Korean BBQ chicken, tuna melts, chicken fingers, pizza, nut butter & jelly sandwiches, or dozens of other tasty dishes, I'm not missing out on anything by living MacroWise.

I get to snack on nacho chips made from almond protein that tastes better than Doritos. I eat cereal made from pea protein that tastes better than fruity pebbles. And I always look forward to my go-to chocolate bar made from milk protein that tastes better than Snickers! All these delicious foods contain natural ingredients, low sugar, low calories, and the right macros. I don't have a good reason to deviate from the list since I enjoy everything I eat. My kitchen is always stocked with my favorite MacroWise snacks and whole foods to ensure I always have something good to eat. Having lots of tasty options from the MacroWise list makes it simple to stay within your healthy boundaries and lose weight consistently. Committing to the list is essential for developing healthy eating habits and maintaining your goal weight permanently.

After maintaining my initial goal for a year, I assessed my situation and decided to lose 5 more pounds. I had a new number in mind for my self-imposed goal weight, which required me to tighten up to achieve it. When I first began my weight-loss journey, I was eating 5 MacroWise snacks plus 1 MacroWise meal per day. 90 days later, I transitioned into eating 4 MacroWise snacks plus 2 MacroWise meals per day. And once I hit my goal weight, I enjoyed 3 MacroWise snacks plus 3 MacroWise meals per day. For me to lose 5 more pounds, I had to tighten up on my calorie intake and shift back to eating 4 snacks plus 2 meals per day. Losing those last 5 pounds was taking a long time, so I switched to eating 5 snacks plus 1 protein & vegetable meal per day. It takes several days of being in a calorie deficit to get back into fat-burning mode. The last few pounds are always the toughest to lose, so you need to be calorie-conscious and choose your foods wisely during this time.

I knew there was room to cut some additional calories throughout my day, so I made a few simple tweaks to lose the last few pounds. Instead of having Greek yogurt with my cereal, I used unsweetened almond milk. I switched from eating snacks with 250 calories and 25 grams of carbs to eating snacks with 150 calories and 10 grams of carbs. I reduced my protein portions during meals from 9 ounces of steak or dark meat chicken to 7 ounces of fish or white meat chicken. I replaced one of my favorite beverages with water just to drop another 40 calories per day. On some days, I waited 3 hours after waking up before having my first MacroWise snack. And I also increased the time between snacks from 2 ½ hours to 3 hours. Plus, if I was entitled to have one last snack close to bedtime, I would skip it to avoid eating late at night. I made calculated adjustments where I could and reached my new goal weight within 3 months. After maintaining my new number for a while, I slowly increased my calorie and macro allowance, while remaining the watcher of my weight. I went back to eating 4 MacroWise snacks plus 2 MacroWise meals per day, which eventually led to eating 1 to 3 MacroWise snacks plus 2 to 3 MacroWise meals per day.

Maintaining this high level of calorie and macro-awareness enables me to enjoy dining out at restaurants with friends and family. I'm careful to choose items on the menu that are also on the MacroWise list like lean protein and steamed vegetables. Some of my favorites are grilled fish, white meat chicken, filet mignon, broccoli, cauliflower, and sweet peppers. And if I want to enjoy a tasty salad, then I bring my own MacroWise dressing with me to the retaurant. If I want bread with my meal, flavor in my water, or dessert like everyone else, then I make sure to bring those items from the list with me as well. Being macro-wise means that you can have your cake and eat it too, so long as the cake is from the MacroWise list!

Most people consider this ongoing process of structuring what and when you eat a matter of habit. I think it became something much deeper than that for me. When a healthy habit you enjoy doing improves your life, it becomes a healthy lifestyle. You don't have to put much thought into doing it because it's part of your new identity. If you choose to see yourself as a healthy, vibrant person who cares about the way you look and feel, then you will likely persist in making lasting changes. It's easy to install healthy eating habits and lose weight when you stick to the foods on the list and follow the basic rules in this book. It only takes a month to create positive change by eating macro-wise. And once you experience the change, you will naturally embrace the MacroWise lifestyle.

Very few people in this world were given good teachers to show them how to eat right. Along the way, we picked up good eating habits mixed with bad ones. A never-ending flood of seductive advertising, combined with easy access to cheap junk food, corrupted our perception of what is good and bad for us. Plus, every third person we see is overweight, which makes us think it's normal to be fat. As a result, we've been lulled into accepting a lie that being thin is not that simple. We believed this lie and got fat by surrendering to it. But the truth is, being thin really is that simple. If you just do the things you're being taught here, then it's done, and you realize it is that simple and that it always was.

CHAPTER NINE

Why Get Help from a MacroWise Coach?

My niece Jordan once came to Miami for a family visit and stayed at my place. She knew her mother was working as a weight loss coach for some diet-food company and heard I was her new client, but she wasn't optimistic about the diet working. Even though she wanted to lose a little weight herself, she didn't believe the program was sustainable after looking into the company's food and hard rules. She was suspicious of all the soy-based, chemical ingredients in the diet snacks her mom was touting and had zero interest in trying them. Jordan was also convinced the diet didn't allow enough calories to function despite the fact she weighs half of what I weighed and requires less food than me.

When Jordan saw me for the first time after losing 50 pounds in 6 months, she was blown away! She couldn't believe I was able to stay on her mom's diet and lose so much weight. I then explained how I used her mom's program to get started, but the real secret to my success came from finding my own tasty, low-sugar, nutrient-dense foods made from healthy ingredients. Once Jordan saw how good I was eating, she got excited about trying "my program" and begged me to coach her.

My sister Stacey, who was my weight-loss coach, introduced me to the macro-diet. The program required me to buy ultra-processed, portion-con-trolled snacks, exclusively from the diet-food company she represented. She helped me get started by ordering a month's worth of macro-friend-ly snacks from their company's website, which cost over $400. Then, she helped me create a list of essential whole foods to buy at the grocery store. She taught me how to read nutrition labels so I could avoid eating foods that cause weight gain. And she was always available by phone to answer my questions along the way.

Having a coach made the rules of the diet clear, which helped me stay committed. My coach made sure I used various smart tools to stay on track. I purchased an air fryer for making protein and vegetable meals fast and easy, a scale for weighing my food to help maintain a calorie deficit, and another scale for weighing my body once a week to track my progress. After weighing myself, I would text her a photo of my weight so she could record my progress and encourage me. I listened to her advice, made the adjustments, and got results. With help from a coach, I consistently lost 2 ½ pounds every week until I reached my goal weight.

Having real support to guide you through one of the biggest health epidemics of all time is key if you're serious about making lasting changes. Working with a coach empowered me to start the weight-loss process right. And by going through the process, I eventually learned how to do things on my own. I discovered hundreds of healthy, low-calorie macro-wise snacks sold on Amazon and in local grocery stores by many independent food manufacturers. I put together a list of fresh, nutritious whole foods to keep stocked in my kitchen. I figured out how to make some of the most amazing macro-wise meals using a variety of low-sugar, tasty ingredients. Having a coach was instrumental in knowing what was required of me to lose weight. And if I slacked off, my coach was there to wake me up!

To this day, I believe that I'm the most successful client my sister ever coached in terms of someone who lost the most weight, got in the best shape, ate the healthiest, and taught others how to do the same. Working with a coach is not just about losing a bunch of weight. It's about establishing good eating habits and knowing how to maintain a realistic goal weight for life. It's also about changing your perception of what food means to you as a healthy human being. Even more so, it's about owning that perception regardless of the good and bad times that come and go throughout one's life.

When I eventually became a coach, I soon realized that some people don't have the extra money to hire a coach to guide them through the weight-loss process. I understood this fact of life all too well and did everything possible to provide affordable help for everybody. I started by including a lot of valuable information in this book, which doesn't cost you anything. Plus, the new macro-wise foods you buy cost about the same as your old macro-dumb foods, so there's no extra cost there. However, paying for professional coaching is something beyond your everyday expenses and is not affordable for everyone, which is why I came up with a wise solution. I recorded an extensive library of daily instructional videos to guide you through the entire process. I took all the same lessons from my live, one-on-one coaching sessions, and organized them in a simple, linear format that you can watch anytime.

The first video takes you online to order a month's worth of MacroWise snacks. The second video helps you create a list of essential groceries to buy. The third video prepares you to transition into eating your new foods. Each day, there's a new video to learn from that builds on the previous day's lesson. There are 90 daily videos to guide you through the 90-day thin phase. After the first MacroWise phase is complete, you can continue watching new daily videos over the next 6 months that guide you through the next 2 MacroWise phases. There are 270 daily videos total that have been methodically designed to coach you through the entire 9-month process of completing all 3 MacroWise phases. These daily videos are an excellent option for getting valuable support that is comparable to what my clients receive during live coaching sessions.

In addition to the daily coaching videos, you can text-a-coach unlimited questions and get clear, direct answers. Our coaching service gives you 24/7 access to a chat group where you receive one-on-one support from a MacroWise coach via texting. Plus, you share relevant information with people in your chat group, which helps you transition from the thin phase, into the lean phase, and then the healthy phase.

Since MacroWise is a progressive lifestyle program comprised of 3 phases, you should raise the bar as you near your goal weight after completing the first phase. The reality is that most of you will have soft muscles and loose skin after losing a bunch of weight. I don't suggest anyone try to lose weight and get fit at the same time for a couple of reasons. Physical exercise increases your appetite, which isn't conducive to losing weight. Plus, doing both at the same time is overwhelming for most, which can lead to quitting. You want to lose weight with the first MacroWise phase, before getting in shape with the second phase. Our coaching service helps you transition from the first 90-day thin phase into the second 90-day lean phase by showing you how to do a few simple exercises. Finding exercises that you enjoy doing makes the lean phase a real pleasure.

MacroWise takes the same non-extreme, middle-path approach toward exercising and getting in shape as it does with eating and losing weight. There are many types of light exercises you can do regardless of age or physical condition. I like power walking with ankle and wrist weights for improving cardio. I enjoy using resistance bands and jumping on a trampoline to tone my muscles. You can choose whichever exercise you want to start with and our coaching service will help you do it right. As your level of exercise increases, your calorie allowance also increases, which opens the door to many new and exciting food options. The videos address every aspect of this process and guide you every step of the way.

Once you reach your goal weight and start getting in shape, you continue evolving with the lifestyle by transitioning into the third and final MacroWise phase. Much like we advise losing weight before getting in shape, we also advise getting in shape before mastering your health. Once you complete the 90-day lean phase, our coaching service helps you transition into the final 90-day healthy phase by showing you better options for higher living.

The 90-day healthy phase teaches you how to take your nutrition, personal care routine, and overall health to the highest level. The coaching videos reveal super foods available in your local grocery store that contain amazing health benefits. They also show you how to identify toxic ingredients hidden in many foods, drinks, and personal care products that cause disease. You will know precisely which ingredients are bad so you can avoid them, and which are good so you can embrace them. We'll introduce you to incredible, natural health supplements for improving your mental, physical, and emotional well-being. Plus, the instructional videos include special exercises for increasing flexibility, strengthening the core, tightening skin, and increasing energy throughout the day. After completing all 3 MacroWise phases using our 9-month coaching service, you will know the secret to being thin, lean, and healthy. You will apply this valuable knowledge toward elevating your appearance, health, and quality of life forever.

There's a small cost for using our online coaching service. However, the long-term benefits are huge. If you're looking for next-level personalized support, we also offer one-on-one phone coaches to guide you through the entire process and help keep you motivated. The metabolic science behind MacroWise combined with our list of nutritious foods and affordable coaching service makes it simple to achieve your ideal body. MacroWise delivers everything you need to be thin, lean, and healthy. You only get one body in this lifetime and you're solely responsible for taking care of it, so get MacroWise and treat it right!

CHAPTER TEN

The Time Is Always Now

The reason you should decide to get in shape now is because there is no other time than now. Making a plan to lose weight sometime in the future or wishing you acted in the past won't change a thing if you want to be thin in the now. Once you decide to change, the time to act on it is always now because you will always be faced with upholding it. And, remembering the decision you made along with your reason for making it will help you practice it and turn it into a good habit. It took many years of living with bad eating habits to get you here. Fortunately, it only takes a few months of developing good ones to get you out. If you wait too long, time will pass you by along with the opportunity to help yourself. Today is already tomorrow, tomorrow is next week, weeks turn into months and years, and before you know it, life passed by. You might as well make a few, simple adjustments to improve yourself in the now before time passes. That's how you make time serve you instead of being a slave to it.

Some would argue that the real reason for making the decision is for something more tangible, like your looks, health, or family. Of course, those are all great reasons. However, the essential reason for deciding to get in shape now is time. We all want to look good, feel great, and enjoy our time with friends and family now before it's too late. But, wanting will not change a thing until you decide that the time to do it is always now. The time is now once you lose 20% of the weight. The time is now once you're halfway there. The time is now once you reach your goal weight. And the time is now after you've maintained your goal weight for a year and have suddenly gained 5 pounds. The time is always now once you decide because that decision requires ongoing maintenance.

I maintained my goal weight for a year before I slipped and gained 5 pounds out of nowhere. Well, at least that's what I thought until I decided to start counting calories again, which revealed the real reason. Simply put, I was overeating and choosing not to count my calories like I used to. I got a little too comfortable with my success and started losing touch with what my lifestyle required. Fortunately, I woke up, got mad, and tightened up after only gaining 5 pounds. It's a slippery slope that can easily turn into a lot more if you don't wake yourself up and make the necessary adjustments. I'm dedicated to maintaining my best body for life because that's the life I chose. I want to look good, feel my best, and enjoy a long, healthy life now. If I waited any longer to make the decision, I'm sure I would have woken up as an obese, sick, 50-year-old man asking the question, "What happened?" I refuse to be that person, which is why I decided to lose weight and get in shape once I found a good plan for doing so.

About 3 months after starting my sister's macro-diet, I bumped into an old friend of mine on the beach who was overweight. We both gained a lot of weight over the years and had previously spoken about wanting to get in shape. Before starting my diet, I told him that I found a good plan for losing weight and made the decision to do it. When he saw the results that I was having after just 3 months, he asked me to help him lose weight too. So, I introduced him to my sister who got him started by ordering a month's worth of protein snacks from the diet food company she represented. Plus, she helped him put together a list of essential groceries to buy. He didn't like the idea of eating ultra-processed, soy-protein snacks, which is one of the reasons why it didn't work for him. Soon after he quit my sister's macro-diet, I showed him some of the healthy, wise-processed snacks and fresh whole foods I discovered, which got him interested again. He asked me to email him my list of foods so he could "take a look at it", but I sensed he wasn't serious about changing, so I didn't bother sending it.

A year flew by and once again I bumped into that same, old friend on the beach, except this time he looked obese and sick while I looked lean and healthy. He was excited to tell me about a new, extreme exercise program he recently signed up for online. He saw an advertisement on YouTube from some fitness guru claiming that you could look like him if you follow his program. So, he signed up and paid the $100 monthly subscription fee, which made him feel obligated to start "just as soon as the holidays are over." I didn't want to discourage him from taking action, but the truth is, he wasn't going to commit to any exercise program after being fat and lazy for most of his life. It's not a practical solution for him or anyone wanting to lose weight permanently after years of living a gluttonous, sedentary lifestyle. From my experience, most people need to go through a gradual process if they want to be realistic about making lasting change.

MacroWise is a progressive lifestyle program comprised of 3 phases, methodically designed to take you through the gradual process of being thin, lean, and healthy. The first phase focuses on losing weight, which is the plan behind this first book, *The Secret To Being Thin*. This 90-day phase replaces high-sugar, nutrient-poor foods with low-sugar, nutrient-rich foods. After developing healthy eating habits and experiencing rapid weight loss, you will be ready to take the next step. The second phase focuses on getting in shape, which is the plan behind the second book, *The Secret To Being Lean*. This next 90-day phase introduces you to simple exercises, like power walking and light resistance training. Your body will start to look and feel better after a few months of exercising. Plus, you get to eat more food since your calorie allowance increases. Once you see your body becoming leaner and stronger, you will be ready to take the last step. The third phase focuses on improving your health, which is the plan behind the third book, *The Secret To Being Healthy*. This final 90-day phase teaches you about next-level nutrition, health supplements, and physical exercises that are intended to elevate your mind, body, and soul. The MacroWise lifestyle starts with losing body fat before building muscles. Then, you can enhance your health by developing a self-care routine that improves your well-being and quality of life. Trying to do it all from the start is too overwhelming and causes a person to quit.

If your weight-loss plan is not something you can live with long-term, then you will eventually give up and gain back the weight. That includes all the people who try to lose weight by going on various extreme "diets", like high-fat or low-fat diets. Or for those who rely on all-meat or liquid diets as their main source of nourishment. Not to mention all the pre-packaged meal programs and calorie counting apps, which promise easy results with minimal effort. And there's no pharamacutical drug or exercise guru in the world that can help you if you don't have a simple plan to eat right for life. If the program you choose for losing weight is unsustainable, then you're just wasting your time and money. You may lose some weight along the way, but you will eventually gain it all back again. And sadly, the only thing that changed was time passing by. If you're serious about losing weight, then you should choose a vehicle that can get you where you want to be and keep you there for good.

Soon after my weight loss journey began, people saw my success and asked me for advice. Once I explained how I ate, they wanted me to give them a list of foods to buy so they could follow my replacement method and lose weight too. I received text messages regularly requesting to send "the list." So, I made a promise to type up my list and email it to them when it was ready. I was inspired to invest my time and effort into creating MacroWise once I knew it could help people. Over time, one thing led to another and MacroWise was born. At the end of the day, I can give you a good plan for losing weight, but I can't make you do it. I can give you the secret to being thin, lean, and healthy, but I can't be there to enforce it. I can provide you with a wellness program that works for life, but the will to actualize it must come from you.

Everything you need to practice the secret to being thin is in this book and on our website. You can achieve great success by going through the book and making it happen on your own. For those of you who tried various diet plans in the past and are discouraged from doing this alone, take a leap of faith by getting professional help from our coaching services. They provide valuable support and empower you to stop wasting precious time since time is the one thing you never get back.

At this point, you have everything you need to make it happen for yourself. There's no room for excuses since you now have a good plan that works, and the support to actualize it. Time is going to fly by, which is why you should decide to get in shape now. If not now, then when? Yesterday is history, tomorrow is a mystery, and today is a gift of life, which is why we call it the present. MacroWise is your gift for replacing bad with good and choosing life. The time to wake up, tighten up, and live up your best life, is now. Do not put it off another day because the time is always now!

CHAPTER ELEVEN

MacroWise Rules

Sugar is your enemy!

The first 72 hours will be the most difficult as your body detoxes from an addictive drug called sugar. Be aware that any pain and cravings you experience are sugar withdrawal symptoms and will pass within a few days.

1st Phase - 5 & 1 Thin

1st 90 Days or Until Goal Weight Reached
(Duration: Up to 3 Months)

- 1,000 to 1,300 calories per day allowance
- Eat 6X a day every 2 ½ hours from the MacroWise list
  - 5 MacroWise snacks
  - 1 MacroWise meal w/ 5-8 oz protein & 5-8 oz vegetables
- 100-125g of protein, 50-100g of carbohydrates, & 25-75g of fat
- Drink 8+ tall glasses of water per day (½-1 gallon)
- Walking 30+ min/day, 3+ days/week is suggested but not necessary

*2nd Phase - 4 & 2 Lean *

After 90 Days or Goal Weight Reached
(Duration: 3+ Months)

- 1,300 to 1,700 calories per day allowance
- Eat 6X a day every 2 ½ hours from the MacroWise list
  - 4 MacroWise snacks

- 2 MacroWise meals w/ protein, fruits, & vegetables
- 100-150g of protein, 75-125g of carbohydrates, & 50-100g of fat
- Drink 8+ tall glasses of water per day (½-1 gallon)
- Walking +/or other exercise 45 min/day, 4+ days/week is mandatory (*increasing your calorie allowance depends on level of exercise, gender, & height*)

3rd Phase - 3 & 3 Healthy
After Lean Phase or Goal Weight Reached
(Duration: For Life)

- 1,500 to 2,300 calories per day
- Eat 4X to 6X a day every 2 ½ to 3 hours from the MacroWise list
  - 1 to 3 MacroWise snacks
  - 2 to 3 MacroWise meals w/ protein, fruits, & vegetables
- 125-150g+ of protein, 75-125g of carbohydrates, & 75-125g of fat
- Drink 8 glasses of purified water per day (½ gallon+)
- Walking +/or other exercise 45 min/day, 4+ days/week is strongly recommended (*ask a MacroWise coach to help you assess & calculate your specific calorie allowance*)

1st Phase - 5 & 1 Thin

- 1,000 to 1,300 calories per day allowance
- Eat your first MacroWise snack within 1 hour of waking up
- Start your phone's timer to remind you to eat 6X a day every 2 ½ hours
- The average number of calories per MacroWise snack is 150
- The maximum number of calories per MacroWise snack is 200
- Any MacroWise snack over 200 calories is a MacroWise meal
- A MacroWise snack must have 10g of protein min, 20g of carbs max, & 15g fat max
- Average carbs per MacroWise snack is 15g, average fat per MacroWise snack is 10g
- A MacroWise meal must have 30g of protein min, 20g of carbs max, &

20g of fat max
- Purchase your favorite go-to items for enjoying MacroWise snacks & meals:
  - Essential Groceries: Low-fat Greek yogurt, cottage cheese, almond milk, eggs, cheese, tuna, bread, jelly, berries, vegetables, tofu, fish, chicken, marinades, condiments, etc.
  - MacroWise snacks: Cereals, bars, chips, puffs, seeds, crackers, soups, shakes, desserts, beverages, etc.

Refer to the "Thin" options on "The List" for choosing essential groceries, snacks, quick meals, smart tools, & other items to help you succeed!

CHAPTER TWELVE

Medical Disclaimer

The Company ("We") recommends that you consult your healthcare provider before starting any weight loss program and during your weight loss program. Do NOT use the MacroWise plan if you are pregnant or under the age of 13.

Before starting a weight loss program, talk with your healthcare provider about the program and about any medications or dietary supplements you are using, including Coumadin (Warfarin), lithium, diuretics, or medications for diabetes, high blood pressure, or thyroid conditions. Do not participate in any MacroWise Program until you are cleared by your healthcare provider if you have or have had a serious illness (e.g., cardiovascular disease including heart attack, diabetes, cancer, thyroid disease, liver, or kidney disease, eating disorders, such as anorexia or bulimia), or any other condition requiring medical care or that may be affected by weight loss.

The MacroWise 5 & 1-Thin Plan is NOT appropriate for teens, sedentary older adults (65 years and older), nursing mothers, people with gout, some people with diabetes, and those who exercise more than 45 minutes per day – if you fall into one of these categories, please consult your healthcare provider and refer to www.MacroWise.com to talk with a MacroWise Coach about other MacroWise plans that may be appropriate. For special medical or dietary needs, including food allergies, consult your healthcare provider and talk to a MacroWise Coach. Do not consume a product if you are allergic to any of the product's ingredients that are listed on the product packaging.

We recommend drinking at least 64 ounces of water each day but not more than 1 gallon. Consult with your healthcare provider before changing the amount of water you drink as it can affect certain health conditions and medications.

NOTE: Rapid weight loss may cause gallstones, gallbladder disease, or temporary hair thinning in some people. While adjusting to the intake of a lower calorie level and dietary changes, some people may experience dizziness, lightheadedness, headache, fatigue, or gastrointestinal disturbances (such as abdominal pain, bloating, gas, constipation, diarrhea, or nausea). Consult your healthcare provider for further guidance on these or any other health concerns. Seek immediate medical attention if you experience muscle cramps, tingling, numbness, confusion, or rapid/irregular heartbeat as these may be a sign of a more serious health condition.

For the avoidance of doubt, the MacroWise Programs, products, and services are not labeled, advertised, or promoted for any specific medicinal purpose, i.e., cure, treatment, or prevention, implied or otherwise, of any disease or disorder, including its related conditions.

The MacroWise Programs, products, and any of its materials and/or information do not in any way constitute medical advice or substitute for medical treatment. As individuals may have different responses to dietary products or changes in diet, consult with your healthcare provider regarding any medical concerns.

For further information regarding this Medical Disclaimer, contact Nutrition Support via email: info@MacroWise.com.

Welcome to MacroWise!

CHAPTER THIRTEEN

Tips to Remember Going into This

- Being thin feels better than food tastes. Fortunately, MacroWise tastes great, satiates, never gets boring, is healthy, and saves you time & money!
- The 1ˢᵗ 90 days are the "5 & 1-Thin Phase". Each day you eat 5 MacroWise snacks plus 1 MacroWise meal that consists of 5 to 8 oz protein & 5 to 8 oz vegetables.
- A MacroWise snack containing 10+ grams of protein will satisfy your body's needs for 2 ½ hours. Do not think otherwise! Eat your snack and know that in a few minutes, you will realize that you're no longer hungry. <u>Stick to the items on the list</u>, <u>eat slowly</u>, <u>be patient</u>, <u>and your hunger will quickly subside</u>.
- Your final MacroWise snack of the night should contain fewer calories, carbs, and fat than any of your previous snacks that same day.
- Make sure to stop eating at least 2 ½ hours before bedtime.
- Tighten up on calories and carbs, & increase protein for faster weight loss.
- Total intake of macros including all meals and snacks cannot exceed daily allowance.
- Pay attention to the serving size of each item to stay within your allowance.
- You may consume any foods you want off the list provided it has

the same nutritional value and macro ratio as the curated foods on the list. (calories - protein/carbs/fat)

- Drink a lot of WATER. Drink at least 1 glass with every MacroWise snack and meal. ½ to 1 gallon of water daily is suggested to digest nutrient-dense foods.
- Drinking more than a ½ gallon of water spread out evenly throughout the day will help you feel full.
- Weigh yourself once a week upon waking up, after you urinate, and before you eat or drink anything to accurately track your weight-loss progress.
- As you reach your goal weight, try not to judge or "fat-shame" people. Just because you chose to improve yourself, doesn't mean others have to.
- Use the MacroWise coaching service to help you create lasting change.

CHAPTER FOURTEEN

What to Avoid

- **Sugar** – check ingredients on all packaging to avoid hidden sugars, fructose, high fructose corn syrup, honey, syrup, etc.
- **Alcohol** - some alcohol is allowed if you stay within your daily calorie allowance but it is not recommended during the 90-day thin phase
- **Sugary Sodas** – replace dirty soda pop with clean soda options on the list
- **Diet Sodas & Drinks** - replace artificial sweeteners with natural ingredients
- **Fruit** - only 4 types of berries are allowed - strawberries, blueberries, blackberries, & raspberries
- **Fruit Juice** – orange, apple, pineapple, grape, mango, cranberry, cherry, etc.
- **Condiments** – only macro-wise condiments from the list are allowed
- **Bread** – only low-carb breads from the list are allowed
- **Grains** – wheat, white & brown rice, pasta, corn, rye, barley, oats, etc.
- **Potatoes & Yams** – stick to low-calorie, low-carb vegetables on the list
- **Oils** – avocado, coconut, and olive oil are allowed in small amounts, but it's best to avoid all cooking oil, and use non-stick

cooking oil spray instead

- **Fatty Foods** – stick to low-cal, low-fat foods during the 90-day thin phase
- **Fried Foods** – only air-fried foods are allowed
- **Fast Food** – only MacroWise snacks and quick meals from the list are allowed
- **Exercise** – walking is suggested but not necessary
- **Negative People** – use the MacroWise coaching service to get the daily support you need from a community of positive, like-minded individuals

CHAPTER FIFTEEN

7-Day Sample Menu

All items in this sample menu are tagged as "Thin" items under their corresponding categories on the list. You get to choose from a large variety of both wise-processed as well as fresh foods. The list offers many vegan, organic, gluten-free, kosher, plant, dairy, fish, chicken, and meat options to fit any lifestyle. There are plenty of inexpensive whole foods, like tofu, tuna, eggs, chicken, and turkey, for keeping your daily food budget under $20. Plus, there are more expensive whole foods, like shrimp, wild-caught salmon, sea bass, and sirloin steak, for larger budgets. After the 90-Day Thin Phase, your calorie and macro allowance will increase, which means more options and larger portions. The MacroWise coaching videos share amazing recipes for making fast, tasty snacks and meals at home. The videos can help you find your favorite low-sugar, nutrient-dense items that fit your budget, so you can design a macro-wise menu that works for you. We made it simple, convenient, and affordable, for anyone to get MacroWise and lose weight permanently!

Monday

- **1st MacroWise snack: Cereal w/ almond milk & coffee**
  1 cup Magic Spoon fruity cereal, w/ 1 cup MOOALA unsweetened organic almond milk, & 1 cup Jacobs instant coffee, mixed w/ 1 tsp Laird mocha coffee creamer
- **Nutrition Facts & Cost:**
  * Cereal: 150 calories 13g protein, 15g carbs, and 7g fat = Cost:

$1.50
* Almond milk: 40 calories, 2g protein, 2g carbs, and 3.5g fat = Cost: $1
* Coffee: 0 calories, 0g protein, 0g carbs, and 0g fat = Cost: $0.25
* Coffee creamer: 10 calories, 0g protein, 1g carbs, and 0.5g fat = Cost: $0.10
- **Total Nutrition Facts & Cost**: 200 calories, 15g protein, 18g carbs, 11g fat. Cost: $2.85

- **2nd MacroWise snack: 5.3 oz Two Good peach-flavored yogurt & 1 glass of water**
  - **Total Nutrition Facts & Cost:** 80 calories, 12g protein, 4g carbs, and 2g fat = Cost: $1.50

- **3rd MacroWise snack: 1 Misfits cookie dough protein bar & 1 glass of water**
  - **Total Nutrition Facts & Cost:** 190 calories, 15g protein, 16g carbs, and 10g fat = Cost: $1.50

- **4th MacroWise snack: 2 large Eggland's Best organic hardboiled eggs, & 1 slice of Sargento ultra-thin Swiss cheese, & 1 glass of water**
  - **Nutrition Facts & Cost**:
    * Eggs: 120 calories, 12g protein, 0g carbs, and 8g fat = Cost: $0.75
    * Cheese: 40 calories, 3g protein, 1g carbs, and 3g fat = Cost: $0.20
  - **Total Nutrition Facts & Cost:** 160 calories, 15g protein, 1g carbs, and 11g fat = Cost: $0.95

- **1 MacroWise meal: Air-fried BBQ Chicken Breast w/ Broccoli, & 1 mango-lemon frozen Popsicle**

8 oz (pre-cooked) boneless skinless chicken breast, w/ 3 tbsp G Hughes BBQ sauce, & 6 ounces (pre-cooked) broccoli w/ 1 tsp sea salt, & 1 DeeBee's Freezie Pop & 1 glass of water

- **Nutrition Facts & Cost**:
  - * Chicken: 250 calories, 48g protein, 0g carbs, and 2g fat = Cost: $4.00
  - * BBQ sauce: 15 calories, 0g protein, 3g carbs, and 0g fat = Cost: $0.37
  - * Broccoli: 30 calories, 2.5g protein, 6g carbs, and 0.3g fat = Cost: $3.50
  - * Salt: 0 calories 0g protein, 0g carbs, and 0.5g fat = Cost: $0.02
  - * Popsicle: 25 calories, 0g protein, 6g carbs, and 0g fat = Cost: $0.54
  - **Total Nutrition Facts & Cost**: 320 calories, 50.5g protein, 15g carbs, 2.8g fat. Cost: $8.43

- **5th MacroWise snack: 1 Better Than Good salted caramel protein puffs & 1 glass of water**
  Total Nutrition Facts & Cost: 110 calories, 16g protein, 4g carbs, and 3.5g fat = Cost: $2.50

Daily Total Nutrition Facts:
1,060 calories, 123.5g protein, 58g carbs, 40.3g fat

Daily Total Cost:
$17.73

Tuesday

- **1st MacroWise snack: Scrambled egg whites w/ cheese & coffee**
  1/2 cup Pete & Gerry's organic egg whites scrambled, w/ 1 slice

Edam light cheese, 1 glass of water, 1 cup of Jacob's instant coffee, mixed w/ 1 scoop of Natural Force marine collagen protein powder & 1 tsp Laird mocha coffee creamer

- **Nutrition Facts & Cost**:
  - * Eggs: 75 calories, 15g protein, 0g carbs, and 0g fat = Cost: $2
  - * Cheese: 60 calories, 8g protein, 0g carbs, and 2.5g fat = Cost: $1.25
  - * Coffee: 0 calories, 0g protein, 0g carbs, and 0g fat = Cost: $0.25
  - * Collagen powder: 45 calories, 10g protein, 0g carbs, and 0g fat = Cost: $1.75
  - * Coffee creamer: 10 calories, 0g protein, 1g carbs, and 0.5g fat = Cost: $0.10
  - **Total Nutrition Facts & Cost:** 190 calories, 33g protein, 1g carbs, and 3g fat = Cost: $5.35

- **2nd MacroWise snack: Cottage cheese & strawberries**
  5.3 oz serving good culture 2% cottage cheese, w/ 6 oz strawberries & 1 glass of water
  - **Nutrition Facts & Cost**:
    - * Ctg. cheese: 120 calories, 19g protein, 3g carbs, and 3g fat = Cost: $2
    - * Strawberries: 54 calories, 1g protein, 12g carbs, and 0.5g fat = Cost: $2.25
    - **Total Nutrition Facts & Cost:** 174 calories, 20g protein, 15g carbs, and 3.5g fat = Cost: $4.25

- **3rd MacroWise snack: 1 Laird lemon almond protein bar & 1 glass of water**
  - **Total Nutrition Facts & Cost:** 180 calories, 10g protein, 19g carbs, and 7g fat = Cost: $2.50

- **4th MacroWise snack: 1 oz People's Choice beef jerky & 1**

can Poppi classic cola

- **Nutrition Facts & Cost:**
    * Jerky: 90 calories, 16g protein, 0g carbs, and 2.5g fat = Cost: $2
    * Soda: 25 calories, 0g protein, 7g carbs, and 0g fat = Cost: $2.25
    - **Total Nutrition Facts & Cost:** 115 calories, 16g protein, 7g carbs, and 2.5g fat = Cost: $4.25

- **1 MacroWise meal: Air-fried sweet chili salmon w/ sweet peppers & 1 glass of water**
  7 oz (pre-cooked) Atlantic salmon, w/ 3 tbsp G Hughes sweet chili sauce, & 6 oz (pre-cooked) sweet peppers, & 1 glass of water
- **Nutrition Facts & Cost:**
    * Salmon: 340 calories, 35g protein, 0g carbs, and 20g fat = Cost: $8
    * Sweet chili sauce: 15 calories, 0g protein, 3g carbs, and 0g fat = Cost: $0.37
    * Sweet peppers: 60 calories, 2g protein, 12g carbs, and 0g fat = Cost: $3.50
    - **Total Nutrition Facts & Cost**: 415 calories, 37g protein, 15g carbs, 20g fat = Cost: $11.87

- **5th MacroWise snack: Perfect Keto mallow munch- chocolate rice crispy bar & 1 glass of water**
    - **Total Nutrition Facts & Cost:** 80 calories, 9g protein, 14g carbs, and 3.5g fat = Cost: $2.50

Daily Total Nutrition Facts:
1,154 calories, 125g protein, 71g carbs, 39.5g fat

Daily Total Cost:
$30.72

Wednesday

- **1st MacroWise snack: Cereal w/ Greek yogurt & coffee**
  1/2 cup Catalina Crunch chocolate cereal, w/ 3/4 cup Fage 0% non-fat plain Greek yogurt, & 1 cup instant black coffee
- **Nutrition Facts & Cost**
  * Cereal: 110 calories, 11g protein, 14g carbs, and 6g fat = Cost: $1.50
  * Yogurt: 90 calories, 18g protein, 5g carbs, and 0g fat = Cost: $1.50
  * Coffee: 0 calories, 0g protein, 0g carbs, and 0g fat = Cost: $0.25
  - **Total Nutrition Facts & Cost**: 200 calories, 29g protein, 19g carbs, 6g fat. Cost: $3.25

- **2nd MacroWise snack: Pizza & lemonade**
  1 large Joseph's Pita, w/ 1/2 cup YO MAMA'S tomato Sauce, w/ 1/4 cup Les Petites-shredded mozzarella cheese, w/ 1 tsp Mc-Cormick- Neapolitan Seasoning, & 1 glass of water, mixed w/ 1 squeeze of Stur lemonade water enhancer
- **Nutrition Facts & Cost:**
  * Pita: 60 calories, 6g protein, 9g carbs, and 1.5g fat = Cost: $0.67
  * Tomato sauce: 60 calories, 1g protein, 5g carbs, and 3.5g fat = Cost: $1.30
  * Cheese: 80 calories, 8g protein, 1g carbs, and 5g fat = Cost: $0.75
  * Seasoning: 0 calories, 0g protein, 0g carbs, and 0g fat = Cost: $0.10
  * Water enhancer: 0 calories, 0g protein, 1g carbs, and 0g fat = Cost: $0.20
  - **Total Nutrition Facts & Cost**: 200 calories, 15g protein, 16g carbs, and 10g fat = Cost: $3.02

- **3rd MacroWise snack:** 1/4 cup Top Fox Snacks organic pop-roasted BBQ flavor pumpkin seeds, & 1 glass of water, mixed w/ 1 tbsp Laird orange guava coconut water powder mix
- **Nutrition Facts & Cost:**
  * Seeds: 160 calories, 10g protein, 4g carbs, and 13g fat = Cost: $1.50
  * Water enhancer: 40 calories, 0g protein, 10g carbs, and 0g fat = Cost: $1
  - **Total Nutrition Facts & Cost:** 200 calories, 10g protein, 14g carbs, and 13g fat = Cost: $2.50

- **4th MacroWise snack:** 2 large Eggland's Best organic hardboiled eggs, & 1 Polly-O- mozzarella string cheese, & 1 glass of water
- **Nutrition Facts & Cost:**
  * Eggs: 120 calories, 12g protein, 0g carbs, and 8g fat = Cost: $0.75
  * Cheese: 80 calories, 7g protein, 1g carbs, and 5g fat = Cost: $0.50
  - **Total Nutrition Facts & Cost:** 200 calories, 19g protein, 1g carbs, and 13g fat = Cost: $1.25

- **1 MacroWise meal:** Tuna salad & crackers w/ vegetable pouch & 1 glass of water
  5 oz can Wild Plant wild tuna, mixed w/ 1 tbsp Hellman's light mayo, mixed w/ lemon juice, sea salt, pepper, & 10 BRAD's crackers everything veggie crisps, & 1 pouch Kekoa Foods beets, fennel, & kale vegetable puree, & 1 glass of water
- **Nutrition Facts & Cost:**
  * Tuna: 150 calories, 33g protein, 0g carbs, and 1g fat = Cost: $4.00
  * Mayonnaise: 35 calories, 0g protein, 1g carbs, and 3.5g fat =

Cost: $0.18

* Vegetable pouch: 50 calories, 3g protein, 12g carbs, and 0g fat = Cost: $2.50

* Lemon, salt & pepper: 0 calories, 0g protein, 0g carbs, and 0.5g fat = Cost: $0.08

* Crackers: 90 calories, 3g protein, 7g carbs, and 6g fat = Cost: $1.50

- **Total Nutrition Facts & Cost**: 325 calories, 39g protein, 20g carbs, 11g fat. Cost: $8.26

- **5th MacroWise snack: 1 Sinless- marsh mallow krisp protein bar, & 1 cup CRETORS cheddar cheese popcorn, & 1 glass of water**
- **Nutrition Facts & Cost:**
  * Bar: 80 calories, 9g protein, 13g carbs, and 3.5g fat = Cost: $3
  * Popcorn: 90 calories, 2g protein, 5g carbs, and 6.5g fat = Cost: $0.35
  - **Total Nutrition Facts & Cost:** 170 calories, 11g protein, 18g carbs, and 10g fat = Cost: $3.35

Daily Total Nutrition Facts:
1,295 calories, 123g protein, 88g carbs, 63g fat

Daily Total Cost:
$21.63

Thursday

- **1st MacroWise snack: Cereal w/ almond milk & coffee**
  1 cup Magic Spoon cocoa cereal, w/ 1 cup Silk 30 unsweetened almond milk, & 1 cup Sun Alchemy mushroom coffee packet, mixed w/ 1 tbsp Nutpods pumpkin spice creamer
- **Nutrition Facts & Cost:**

* Cereal: 140 calories, 13g protein, 15g carbs, and 7g fat = Cost: $1.50
* Almond milk: 30 calories, 1g protein, 1g carbs, and 2.5g fat = Cost: $0.75
* Coffee: 3 calories, 0g protein, 0g carbs, and 0g fat = Cost: $1
* Coffee creamer: 10 calories, 0g protein, 0g carbs, and 1g fat = Cost: $0.10
- **Total Nutrition Facts & Cost**: 183 calories, 14g protein, 16g carbs, 10.5g fat. Cost: $3.35

- **2nd MacroWise snack: PB&J sandwich & sweet iced tea**
  1 medium Joseph's Pita, w/ 3 tbsp PB2 powdered peanut butter, w/ 1 tbsp GOOD GOOD strawberry jelly, & 1 can Swoon sweet iced tea, mixed with 1 glass of water
- **Nutrition Facts & Cost:**
    * Pita: 50 calories, 5g protein, 7g carbs, and 1.5g fat = Cost: $0.50
    * Peanut butter mix: 90 calories, 9g protein, 7g carbs, and 2.5g fat = Cost: $0.30
    * Jelly: 5 calories, 0g protein, 5g carbs, and 6g fat = Cost: $0.35
    * Iced tea: 5 calories, 0g protein, 1g carbs, and 0g fat = Cost: $2
- **Total Nutrition Facts & Cost**: 150 calories, 14g protein, 20g carbs, and 10g fat = Cost: $3.15

- **3rd MacroWise snack: 1 Feel Vegan mint chocolate chip protein bar & 1 glass of water**
  - **Total Nutrition Facts & Cost:** 200 calories, 15g protein, 12g carbs, and 10g fat = Cost: $3

- **4th MacroWise snack: 1 oz bag Quevos egg white cheddar chips, & 2/3 cup Arctic Zero chocolate ice cream, & 1 glass of water**
- **Nutrition Facts & Cost:**
    * Chips: 120 calories, 8g protein, 9g carbs, and 7g fat = Cost: $2

* Ice cream: 50 calories, 2g protein, 11g carbs, and 0g fat = Cost: $1.75
- **Total Nutrition Facts & Cost:** 170 calories, 10g protein, 20g carbs, and 7g fat = Cost: $3.75

- **1 MacroWise meal: Baked BBQ chicken w/ cauliflower & strawberry Jell-O & 1 glass orange water**
  10 oz Kevin's Korean BBQ-style chicken, w/ 6 oz cauliflower, & 1 cup strawberry Jell-O & 2 glasses water, mixed w/ 2 packets True- orange flavor water enhancer
  - **Nutrition Facts & Cost:**
    * Chicken: 300 calories 46g protein, 10g carbs, and 8g fat = Cost: $6.50
    * Cauliflower: 30 calories, 2g protein, 5g carbs, and 0.3g fat = Cost: $3
    * Jell-O: 10 calories, 1g protein, 0g carbs, and 0g fat = Cost: $0.80
    * Water enhancer: 0 calories, 0g protein, 1g carbs, and 0g fat = Cost: $0.25
  - **Total Nutrition Facts & Cost:** 340 calories, 49g protein, 16g carbs, 8.3g fat. Cost: $10.55

- **5th MacroWise snack: 1 packet WonderSlim- creamy protein cheesecake & 1 glass of water**
  - **Total Nutrition Facts & Cost:** 120 calories, 12g protein, 8g carbs, and 4.5g fat = Cost: $2.50

Daily Total Nutrition Facts:
1,163 calories, 114g protein, 92g carbs, 50.3g fat.

Daily Total Cost:
$26.30

Friday

- <u>1st MacroWise snack</u>: **Cottage cheese w/ blackberries, blueberries & coffee**
  5.3 oz Good Culture 2% cottage cheese, w/ 3 oz blackberries, 2 oz blueberries & 1 cup instant coffee, mixed w/ 1 tbsp Nutpods pumpkin spice coffee creamer
- **Nutrition Facts & Cost**:
    * Ctg. cheese: 120 calories, 19g protein, 3g carbs, and 3g fat = Cost: $2
    * Blackberries: 37 calories, 0.5g protein, 8g carbs, and 0g fat = Cost: $2.00
    * Blueberries: 30 calories, 0.5g protein, 8g carbs, and 0g fat = Cost: $1.50
    * Coffee: 0 calories, 0g protein, 0g carbs, and 0g fat = Cost: $0.25
    * Coffee creamer: 10 calories, 0g protein, 0g carbs, and 1g fat = Cost: $0.10
    - **Total Nutrition Facts & Cost:** 197 calories, 20g protein, 19g carbs, and 4g fat = Cost: $5.85

- <u>2nd MacroWise snack</u>: **Chicken salad w/ chips & 1 glass peach mango flavored water**
  2.6 oz pouch StarKist chicken salad, & 1 oz bag Kibo ranch lentil chips, & 1 glass of water, mixed with 1 IQMIX- peach mango water enhancer powder packet
- **Nutrition Facts & Cost**:
    * Chicken: 70 calories, 10g protein, 4g carbs, and 1.5g fat = Cost: $2
    * Chips: 110 calories, 6g protein, 14 carbs, and 3.5g fat = Cost: $1.50
    * Water enhancer: 10 calories, 0g protein, 1g carbs, and 0g fat = Cost: $1
    - **Total Nutrition Facts & Cost**: 190 calories, 16g protein, 19g

carbs, 5g fat. Cost: $4.50

- **3rd MacroWise snack**: 1 Polly-O mozzarella string cheese, & 1 KILLER vanilla ice cream sandwich, & 1 glass of water
  - **Nutrition Facts & Cost:**
    * Cheese: 80 calories, 7g protein, 1g carbs, and 5g fat = Cost: $0.50
    * Ice cream: 120 calories, 5g protein,14g carbs, and 9g fat = Cost: $1.50
    - **Total Nutrition Facts & Cost:** 200 calories, 12g protein, 15g carbs, and 14g fat = Cost: $2

- **1 MacroWise meal**: **Plant-Based ground burger wrap w/ asparagus & lemonade**
  5 oz Everything Legendary plant-based ground, w/ 1 Egglife egg white everything wrap, w/ 1 tbsp YO MAMMA'S ketchup, 1 tbsp Gulden's- spicy brown mustard, w/ 1 handful shredded lettuce, w/ 2 slices of tomato, & 6 oz (pre-cooked) asparagus, & 1 glass of water, mixed w/ 1 squeeze of SweetLeaf organic monk fruit lemonade water enhancer
  - **Nutrition Facts & Cost**:
    * Ground: 300 calories, 32g protein, 9g carbs, and 13g fat = Cost: $3.50
    * Wrap: 35 calories, 6g protein, 1g carbs, and 1g fat = Cost: $0.65
    * Lettuce & tomato: 10 calories, 1g protein, 2g carbs, and 0g fat = Cost: $0.35
    * Ketchup: 0 calories 1g protein, 1g carbs, and 0g fat = Cost: $0.25
    * Mustard: 5 calories 0g protein, 0g carbs, and 0g fat = Cost: $0.05
    * Asparagus: 30 calories 2g protein, 5g carbs, and 0.5g fat =

Cost: $2.50

* Water enhancer: 0 calories 0g protein, 0g carbs, and 0g fat = Cost: $0.07

- **Total Nutrition Facts & Cost**: 380 calories, 42g protein, 18g carbs, 14.5g fat. Cost: $7.37

- <u>**4th MacroWise snack**</u>: **1 bottle Fuel For Fire vegan mango coconut smoothie squeeze pouch**
  - **Total Nutrition Facts & Cost:** 120 calories, 10g protein, 17g carbs, and 0.5g fat = Cost: $2.50

- <u>**5th MacroWise snack**</u>: **1 Better Than Good strawberries & cream protein puffs & 1 glass of water**
  - **Total Nutrition Facts & Cost:** 130 calories, 14g protein, 4g carbs, and 4.5g fat = Cost: $3

Daily Total Nutrition Facts:

1,217 calories, 114g protein, 92g carbs, 42.5g fat

Daily Total Cost:

$25.22

Saturday

- <u>**1st MacroWise snack**</u>: **cereal w/ almond milk & coffee**
  1 cup: ratio KETO vanilla almond crunch cereal, w/ 1 cup Silk 30 unsweetened almond milk, & 1 cup instant coffee, mixed w/ 1 tbsp Nutpods toasted marshmallow creamer
- **Nutrition Facts & Cost**:
  * Cereal: 140 calories, 10g protein, 19g carbs, and 7g fat = Cost: $1.50
  * Almond milk: 30 calories, 1g protein, 1g carbs, and 2.5g fat = Cost: $0.75

* Coffee: 0 calories, 0g protein, 0g carbs, and 0g fat = Cost: $0.25
* Coffee creamer: 10 calories, 0g protein, 0g carbs, and 1g fat = Cost: $0.10
- **Total Nutrition Facts & Cost**: 180 calories, 11g protein, 20g carbs, 10.5g fat. Cost: $2.60

- **2nd MacroWise snack: 5.3 oz OIKOS PRO mixed berry flavored yogurt & 1 glass of water**
  - **Total Nutrition Facts & Cost:** 140 calories, 20g protein, 8g carbs, and 3g fat = Cost: $1.80

- **3rd MacroWise snack: 1 oz bag Hilo Life nacho tortilla chips & 1 cup Folgers instant coffee, mixed w/ Natural Force marine collagen protein powder**
  - **Nutrition Facts & Cost:**
    *Chips: 150 calories, 9g protein, 5g carbs, and 10g fat = Cost: $1.50
    * Coffee: 0 calories, 0g protein, 0g carbs, and 0g fat = Cost: $0.25
    * Collagen powder: 45 calories, 10g protein, 0g carbs, and 0g fat = Cost: $1.75
  - **Total Nutrition Facts & Cost:** 195 calories, 19g protein, 5g carbs, and 10g fat = Cost: $3.50

- **4th MacroWise snack: 1 IQ banana nut protein bar & 1 glass of water**
  - **Total Nutrition Facts & Cost:** 180 calories, 12g protein,11g carbs, and 14g fat = Cost: $2

- **1 MacroWise meal: Sliced turkey breast w/ gravy & cauliflower stir fry rice & iced tea**
  8 oz Jennie-O boneless turkey breast, w/ 1/4 cup HEINZ gravy,

& 4 oz Tattooed Chef cauliflower stir fry rice, & 1 glass of water, mixed w/ STUR fruit punch water enhancer

- **Nutrition Facts & Cost**:

  * Turkey: 220 calories, 40g protein, 2g carbs, and 2g fat = Cost: $6.75

  * Gravy: 25 calories, 0g protein, 3g carbs, and 1.5g fat = Cost: $0.42

  * Rice: 60 calories, 3g protein, 8g carbs, and 3g fat = Cost: $2

  * Water enhancer: 0 calories, 0g protein, 1g carbs, and 0g fat = Cost: $0.20

  - **Total Nutrition Facts & Cost**: 305 calories, 43g protein, 14g carbs, 6.5g fat. Cost: $9.37

- **5th MacroWise snack: 1 good! - KETO choc. fudge protein bar & 1 glass of water**

  - **Total Nutrition Facts & Cost:** 170 calories, 11g protein, 19g carbs, and 10g fat = Cost: $2

Daily Total Nutrition Facts:

1,170 calories, 116g protein, 77g carbs, 54g fat

Daily Total Cost:

$21.27

Sunday

- **1st MacroWise snack: Peanut chocolate protein bar & coffee**

  1 cold Nick's peanut chocolate bar, w/ 1 cup FOUR SIGMATIC organic mushroom coffee packet, mixed w/ 1 tbsp Nutpods pumpkin spice coffee creamer, & 1 glass of water

- **Nutrition Facts & Cost**:

  * Bar: 190 calories, 15g protein, 20g carbs, and 10g fat = Cost:

$1.75
* Coffee: 0 calories, 0g protein, 0g carbs, and 0g fat = Cost: $1
* Coffee creamer: 10 calories, 0g protein, 0g carbs, and 1g fat = Cost: $0.10
- **Total Nutrition Facts & Cost**: 200 calories, 15g protein, 20g carbs, 11g fat. Cost: $2.85

- **2nd MacroWise snack:** **Egg salad wrap & 1 glass orange clementine water**
  2 large Organic Valley hardboiled eggs, mixed w/ 1 tbsp Hellman's light mayo, mixed w/ a dash of sea salt, pepper, paprika, & shredded lettuce, 2 slices of tomato & 1 Egglife egg white everything wrap, & 1 glass of water, mixed w/ 1 squeeze STUR orange enhancer
- **Nutrition Facts & Cost:**
    * Eggs: 120 calories, 12g protein, 0g carbs, and 8g fat = Cost: $1
    * Mayonnaise: 35 calories, 0g protein, 1g carbs, and 3.5g fat = Cost: $0.18
    * Salt, pepper, & paprika: 0 calories, 0g protein, 0g carbs, and 0g fat = Cost: $0.30
    * Lettuce & tomato: 10 calories, 1g protein, 2g carbs, and 0g fat = Cost: $0.35
    * Wrap: 35 calories, 6g protein, 1g carbs, and 1g fat = Cost: $0.65
    * Water enhancer: 0 calories, 0g protein, 1g carbs, and 0g fat = Cost: $0.20
  - **Total Nutrition Facts & Cost:** 200 calories, 19g protein, 5g carbs, and 12.5g fat = Cost: $2.68

- **3rd MacroWise snack:** **Ramen noodle soup w/ beef bone broth**
  1 packet BARE BONES beef bone broth powder, mixed with 12 oz

hot water, & 3.5 oz package Noodle Revolution ramen style egg white noodles

- **Nutrition Facts & Cost**:
    * Bone Broth: 50 calories, 10g protein, 3g carbs, and 0g fat = Cost: $2
    * Noodles: 45 calories, 10g protein, 1g carbs, and 0g fat = Cost: $4.50
    - **Total Nutrition Facts & Cost:** 95 calories, 20g protein, 4g carbs, and 0g fat = Cost: $6.50

- <u>**4th MacroWise snack**</u>**: 1 Cesar's Kitchen creamy garlic chicken bistro bowl & 1 glass of water**
    - **Total Nutrition Facts & Cost:** 190 calories, 16g protein,14g carbs, and 7g fat = Cost: $5

- <u>**1 MacroWise meal**</u>**: Shrimp alfredo pasta & 1 cherry chia fruit squeeze & 1 glass peach water**
    9 oz jumbo cooked shrimp, w/ 7 oz It's Skinny pasta, mixed w/ 1/2 cup Prego light alfredo sauce, & 1 Mamma Chia cherry love fruit pouch, & 1 glass of water, mixed w/ 1 squeeze of SweetLeaf organic monk fruit orange passionfruit water enhancer
- **Nutrition Facts & Cost**:
    * Shrimp: 180 calories, 33g protein, 0g carbs, and 1.5g fat = Cost: $8
    * Sauce: 90 calories, 2g protein, 6g carbs, and 6g fat = Cost: $0.70
    * Konjac pasta: 60 calories, 3g protein, 4g carbs, and 0g fat = Cost: $3
    * Chia Squeeze: 70 calories, 2g protein, 10g carbs, and 2.5g fat = Cost: $1.25
    * Water enhancer: 0 calories, 0g protein, 0g carbs, and 0g fat = Cost: $0.07
    - **Total Nutrition Facts & Cost**: 400 calories, 40g protein,

20g carbs, 10g fat. Cost: $13.02

- **5th MacroWise snack: Quest Nutrition cheddar cheese crackers & 1 glass of water**
  - **Total Nutrition Facts & Cost:** 130 calories, 10g protein, 10g carbs, and 10g fat = Cost: $1.75

Daily Total Nutrition Facts:
1,215 calories, 120g protein, 73g carbs, 50.5g fat

Daily Total Cost:
$31.80

Designing your own menu is a very important part of the MacroWise life-style. There's a huge variety of good options to choose from on the list, which is why you never get bored. Finding your favorite go-to items on the list and knowing how to make fast, tasty MacroWise meals will take some time and practice. The MacroWise coaching videos expedite this process by sharing amazing recipes for making fresh, nutritious snacks and meals at home. Some of the videos show you how to keep your daily budget under $15. Plus, they expound on the MacroWise rules, which help you stay conscious of your new lifestyle and keep you motivated to pursue it. We made it simple, convenient, and affordable for anyone to get MacroWise and maintain their goal weight for life!

Part 2

The List

Free access at MacroWise.com

CHAPTER SIXTEEN

What Is "The List"?

MacroWise was founded on 2 fundamental principles: Eat the foods from the list 6X a day every 2 ½ hours and stay within your calorie & macro range. "The List" is a curation of foods, beverages, and other macro-wise items containing the right number of calories and macronutrients you need to stay in your weight-loss zone. The list delivers a variety of "Categories", which include essential groceries, MacroWise snacks, fruits & vegetables, marinades & dressings, desserts, beverages, party favors, and more. All items are carefully vetted to ensure they contain healthy, non-GMO ingredients and bring true value. If they don't, then they don't make it onto the list. We enforce a high standard of quality control when choosing items to go on the list.

MacroWise is a progressive lifestyle program comprised of 3 phases to help you lose weight, get in shape, and live a healthy life. The 3 MacroWise "Phases" are defined as: "Phase 1- Thin", "Phase 2- Lean", and "Phase 3- Healthy." Consequently, all foods, beverages, and other items within each category on the list are displayed under 3 sub-categories or phases - "Thin", "Lean", and "Healthy." The items are organized under 3 phases to help you choose the foods that support the phase you're in. Progressing through the phases entitles you to enjoy new levels of delicious, nutritious options on the list as your calorie and macronutrient allowance increases.

The MacroWise list is your gateway to locate and purchase these high-quality, macro-friendly foods from multiple online stores and local grocery stores. The items on the list are displayed with their basic nutrition facts to help you calculate your daily allowance. The list connects you to a world of macro-wise snacks to make it convenient to fuel up 6X a day every 2 ½ hours. "MacroWise snacks" are a fast, tasty, and simple way to get the right number of calories and macronutrients needed to stay satisfied throughout your waking hours. There are hundreds of healthy, pre-packaged, portion-controlled snacks available online at Amazon. Plus, there are lots of tasty, low-sugar, whole foods you can buy at your local grocery store to make your own MacroWise snacks and nutritious meals at home. All the items on the list are linked to multiple online platforms, like Amazon, Instacart, and Whole Foods, so it's easy for you to view, order, and stick to the plan.

Keeping your kitchen stocked with macro-wise foods from the list is essential for staying in your calorie and macro range so you can lose weight permanently. The list saves you a lot of time, effort, and aggravation from worrying about what, when, and where to eat. Plus, it helps you develop healthy eating habits you own for life.

CHAPTER SEVENTEEN

Smart Tools

There are some valuable tools you can utilize to ease your MacroWise 5 & 1- Thin lifestyle. "Smart Tools" is a non-edible category on the list that connects you to a variety of essential items intended to elevate your health and support your weight-loss journey.

Some of the items in this category are common household items that you may already own, like a measuring cup to maintain portion control when making meals or storage containers to keep foods fresh in the fridge. Some items may be new to you, like a vacuum sealer machine for storing individual portions of protein in the freezer or an electric toilet bidet for making your personal care routine a little easier. Some smart tools are free, like an app you download on your phone that reminds you to eat 6X a day every 2 ½ hours. Others cost money but pay dividends for years, like an air fryer for making fast, tasty, nutrient-dense meals. Some of these items are essential for losing weight and getting in shape while others are non-essential but offer convenience and come with various health benefits.

A proper scale for weighing your body once a week is considered an essential item as is a digital scale for weighing your food when making MacroWise snacks and MacroWise meals. Resistance bands are a great option for doing light, anaerobic exercises, like strength training for building muscles and boosting your metabolism. Body weights are good for doing light, aerobic exercises, like walking to burn calories and improving your cardio when you transition into the lean phase. This category also includes some pharmaceutical weight-loss drugs for suppressing your appetite as a non-essential item. We don't advise using drugs since your food cravings will dissipate naturally once sugar leaves your body.

MacroWise does not require you to exercise to lose weight. But after the 90-day thin phase, light exercise is mandatory for achieving the kind of body shape you want. You will likely have flabby muscles and loose skin after losing a bunch of weight. You can fix that by exercising with resistance bands to tone your muscles and by walking with wrist and ankle weights to tighten your body. MacroWise offers online instructional videos to coach you through this next phase if you want professional help. The coaching videos address every aspect of the MacroWise lifestyle as you transition from thin to lean to healthy.

The Smart Tools on the list will ease your weight-loss journey and help you achieve the body you want.

CHAPTER EIGHTEEN

Health Supplements

There are some powerful supplements you can utilize to enhance your MacroWise 5 & 1- Thin lifestyle. "Health Supplements" is a category on the list that connects you to a variety of medicinal items intended to elevate your health and support your weight-loss journey.

Even though the curated foods on the list are rich in both macronutrients and essential micronutrients, there are additional ways to improve your health. During the 90-day rapid weight-loss phase, your calorie allowance is at its lowest point. As a result, you may not be getting enough micronutrients needed to be healthy while losing weight. Micronutrients produce enzymes, hormones, and other substances to improve your health and overall well-being. Micronutrients or "Micros" are commonly referred to as vitamins and minerals, which are associated with improved mood, energy levels, and appetite control. There are 26 essential vitamins and minerals in food that all contribute to endless bodily functions. Correcting even a minor deficiency in a micro can lead to drastic improvements in your health and day-to-day life. This category ensures you get the proper balance of nutrition as you transition through the 3 phases of MacroWise. All the health supplements on the list, including micronutrients, were selected for their ability to support weight-loss, fight disease, and elevate your quality of life.

Some of the items in this category include essential micronutrients, like vitamins A, B6, B12, C, D, E, K, magnesium, calcium, and zinc, which are vital to healthy development, disease prevention, and well-being. And other items, like clean protein powder and MCT oil, help you get the right number of macros while losing weight. Supplements like marine collagen and NAD have anti-aging benefits that improve the appearance of your hair, skin, and nails, while other items, like GABA and L-Tryptophan, help you relax and fall asleep naturally. Many of these health supplements provide a natural alternative to pharmaceutical drugs and have little to no side effects. This category also offers numerous personal care items for elevating your mind and body. Some of these items include aluminum-free deodorant, fluoride-free toothpaste, talc-free baby powder, chemical-free baby wipes, shaving creams, moisturizers, soaps, and shampoos. There's also a variety of natural, non-addictive supplements that can be used for increasing relaxation, mood, and focus as well as decreasing anxiety, stress, and pain.

The Health Supplements on the list were chosen for their ability to advance your weight-loss journey while boosting your mental and physical well-being.

CHAPTER NINETEEN

Marinades, Sauces, Dressings, Condiments,
Spices & Sweeteners

There are many enjoyable flavors you can utilize to uplift your MacroWise 5 & 1-Thin lifestyle. "Marinades, Sauces, Dressings, Condiments, Spices & Sweeteners" is a category on the list that connects you to a variety of low-sugar items intended to elevate your eating experience and support your weight-loss journey.

The tasty items in this category deliver natural, low-calorie, low-carb nutrition without compromising flavor or health. Moving forward, you must find your favorite items for keeping your calorie and macronutrient intake within the correct range. Adding flavor to your food is one of the fastest ways to gain weight without realizing it. Most of the marinades, sauces, dressings, condiments, and sweeteners in the grocery store are either high in sugar, calories, carbs, and fat or full of bad chemicals and artificial sweeteners. Using them will turn a light, macro-wise day into a heavy, macro-dumb lifestyle. This category ensures you choose low-sugar, low-calorie, macro-friendly flavors for making nutrient-dense meals and snacks.

Some of the items in this category are common kitchen items you may already own, such as salt, pepper, cinnamon, cooking oil, mayonnaise, ketchup, mustard, and salad dressing. Spices like salt, pepper, and cinnamon are low in sugar and calories and can remain in your kitchen. However, high-calorie items, like cooking oil, mayo, ketchup, and your favorite salad dressing, will likely have to go. High-fat cooking oil needs to be replaced with fat-free, cooking oil spray. Regular mayonnaise needs to be replaced with light mayo. Regular ketchup needs to be replaced with a sugar-free one, but your current mustard can stay. The wrong dressing can turn your light, macro-friendly salad into the equivalent of a macro-heavy, fast-food meal. You'll need to find a light, natural salad dressing from the list when enjoying a salad.

Just like most items on the list, the options in this category are listed under 3 subcategories called phases to ensure you choose the items that support the phase you're in. By sticking to the items on the list, you get to enjoy guilt-free teriyaki fish, chicken parmesan, sweet & sour tofu, pizza, fajitas, fried chicken, BBQ ribs, shrimp stir fry, and many other tasty MacroWise meals without crossing the macro line.

Regardless of which MacroWise phase you're in, this category delivers quality replacements for all your favorite flavors. The list makes it simple to enjoy the foods you love while staying in your weight-loss zone.

CHAPTER TWENTY

Beverages

There are many tasty drinks you can utilize to enjoy your MacroWise 5 & 1-Thin lifestyle. "Beverages" is a category on the list that connects you to a variety of low-sugar items intended to elevate your drinking experience and support your weight-loss journey.

The refreshing items in this category deliver natural, low-calorie, low-carb nutrition without compromising flavor or health. Moving forward, you must find your favorite items for keeping your calorie and macronutrient intake within the correct range. Drinking regular sodas and juices throughout the day is one of the fastest ways to gain weight without realizing it. Most of the beverages in the grocery store are either, high in sugar, calories, and carbs or full of bad chemicals and artificial sweeteners. Consuming them will turn a light macro-wise day into a heavy, macro-dumb lifestyle. This category ensures you have a wide variety of low-sugar, low-calorie, macro-friendly options to choose from.

Water should always be your drink-of-choice to hydrate, satisfy your thirst, and digest your nutrient-dense snacks. Fortunately, there are lots of tasty, healthy, water enhancers that can transform plain water into your favorite beverage. Some enhancers offer extra hydration and nutrients while others only add flavor. There's also a huge variety of healthy, packaged drinks that will keep you satisfied as well. Some of these natural options include kombucha, iced tea, lemonade, coconut water, hibiscus water, cactus water, sparkling water, sparkling tea, soda pop, prebiotic soda, probiotic soda, mood drinks, vitamin drinks, energy drinks, coffee, green tea, espresso, coffee creamers, and more.

Mainstream drinks loaded with addictive sugar, high-fructose corn syrup, and unhealthy ingredients are replaced with macro-wise drinks made with non-addictive sweeteners, organic fruits, and healthy ingredients. Contents like bisphenol (BPA), artificial colors, phosphoric acid, brominated vegetable oil, sodium benzoate, sucralose, saccharin, aspartame, and acesulfame potassium are replaced with vitamins, electrolytes, sodium, calcium, potassium, natural sweeteners, gluten-free, kosher, vegan, and non-GMO sustainable contents.

Regardless of which MacroWise phase you're in, this category delivers quality replacements for all your favorite beverages. Your options for tasty drinks will expand as you transition from one phase to the next. This category makes it simple to enjoy the beverages you love while staying in your weight-loss zone.

CHAPTER TWENTY-ONE

Fruits & Vegetables

There are many types of nutritious produce you can utilize to enrich your MacroWise 5 & 1-Thin lifestyle. "Fruits & Vegetables" is a category on the list that connects you to a variety of low-sugar items intended to elevate your eating experience and support your weight-loss journey.

The fresh items in this category deliver natural, low-carb, high-fiber nutrition without compromising flavor or health. Moving forward, you must find your favorite items for keeping your calorie and macronutrient intake within the correct range. Snacking on fruits, like mango, cherries, bananas, apples, and grapes, throughout the day is one of the fastest ways to gain weight without realizing it. Most of the fruits in the grocery store are high in sugar, calories, and carbs. Eating them will turn a light, macro-wise day into a heavy, macro-dumb lifestyle. This category ensures you have a variety of low-sugar, low-calorie, macro-friendly options.

During the "90-Day Thin Phase", it's better to avoid fruit altogether because the hidden sugars will kick you out of the fat-burn state and make you feel hungry. You can get your vitamins, minerals, folate, dietary fiber, and other essential nutrients from supplements. However, there is one macro-friendly fruit option you can enjoy during this time - berries! Strawberries, blueberries, blackberries, and raspberries are allowed. You can add 1 cup of berries to cottage cheese or Greek yogurt to enjoy as a MacroWise snack. Strawberries have the fewest carbs of all types of berries while blackberries have the fewest net carbs. They're an excellent source of antioxidants, potassium, and vitamin C among many other nutrients. Plus, berries also contain phytochemicals, which are compounds that may prevent certain chronic diseases.

In addition to eating fruits like berries, vegetables are very important to your health as well. They provide essential vitamins, minerals, antioxidants, and fiber. Fresh vegatables are your best choice, but you can also store frozen ones in the freezer. Each day, you need to add 5 to 8 ounces of vegetables to your protein-of-choice when having your daily MacroWise meal. Your best thin options for vegetables are broccoli, cauliflower, sweet peppers, and asparagus. Wash, marinade, and drop them in the air fryer for 10 minutes along with 5 to 8 ounces of protein. Feel free to add sea salt to the broccoli or hot sauce to the cauliflower for more flavor. There are many fast, tasty ways to enjoy fresh, nutritious produce when making snacks and meals.

Regardless of which MacroWise phase you're in, this category makes it simple to enjoy a healthy balance of nutrition while staying in your weight-loss zone.

CHAPTER TWENTY-TWO

Essential Groceries

There are many satisfying whole foods you can utilize to maintain your MacroWise 5 & 1-Thin lifestyle. "Essential Groceries" is a main category on the list that connects you to a variety of low-sugar items intended to elevate your eating experience and support your weight-loss journey.

The essential items in this category deliver natural, high-protein, low-carb nutrition without compromising flavor or health. Moving forward, you must find your favorite items for keeping your calorie and macronutrient intake within the correct range. Consuming foods that are not on the list is one of the fastest ways to gain weight without realizing it. Most of the foods in the grocery store are high in sugar, calories, carbs, and fat. Eating them will turn a light, macro-wise day into a heavy, macro-dumb lifestyle. This category ensures you have a variety of low-sugar, low-calorie, macro-friendly options, for making your favorite MacroWise snacks and meals.

During the 90-day, 5 & 1-Thin Phase, you eat 5 MacroWise snacks plus 1 MacroWise meal per day consisting of protein & vegetables. Your protein-of-choice should weigh between 5 to 8 ounces depending on the protein source. For example, 5 ounces of steak has the same number of calories as 8 ounces of chicken breast. Your vegetables-of-choice should also weigh 5 to 8 ounces. Since your calorie allowance is between 1,100 to 1,300 for the first 90 days, you must be mindful and make wise choices. It's important to keep your kitchen stocked with an ample supply of your favorite protein for making nutrient-dense meals. You can freeze individual portions of steaks, chicken breasts, ground beef, turkey patties, fish fillets, and veggie burgers to ensure you always have protein for making your daily MacroWise meal. In addition to storing protein in your freezer, you should stock your refrigerator with more protein-rich foods, like low-fat Greek yogurt, low-fat cottage cheese, cheese, lunch meat, tofu, vegan protein, and eggs. Also keep your cabinets stocked with tuna cans, nut butter, cereal, bread, jerky, plant-based burger mix, nuts, and seeds.

Just like most items on the list, the options in this category are listed under 3 subcategories called phases to help you choose the foods that support the phase you're in. By sticking to the macro-wise groceries on the list, you get to enjoy guilt-free fried chicken, tacos, cheeseburgers, chicken fingers, vegatable omelets, tuna melts, pepperoni pizza, almond butter & jelly sandwiches, and plenty more.

Regardless of which MacroWise phase you're in, this category makes it simple to enjoy your favorite foods while staying in your weight-loss zone.

CHAPTER TWENTY-THREE

MacroWise Snacks

There are many amazing foods you can utilize to sustain your MacroWise 5 & 1-Thin lifestyle. "MacroWise snacks" is a main category on the list that connects you to a variety of low-sugar items intended to elevate your eating experience and support your weight-loss journey.

The nourishing items in this category deliver natural, high-protein, low-carb nutrition without compromising flavor or health. Moving forward, you must find your favorite items for keeping your calorie and macronutrient intake within the correct range. Snacking on foods that are not on the list is one of the fastest ways to gain weight without realizing it. Most of the snacks in the grocery store are high in sugar, calories, and carbs. Eating them will turn a light, macro-wise day into a heavy, macro-dumb lifestyle. This category ensures you have a variety of low-sugar, low-calorie, macro-friendly options for fueling up 6 times a day every 2 ½ hours.

There's a popular misconception that processed foods are unhealthy. The fact is, some processed foods, like almond milk, Greek yogurt, cereal, canned fish, nut butters, tofu, frozen fruits & vegetables, hummus, and rotisserie chicken, are just as healthy as whole foods. The same is true for processed, portion-controlled protein snacks. The pre-packaged snacks in this category were selected because they're healthy, tasty, and have a good ratio of macros to ensure you stay satisfied.

Mainstream snacks lacking protein, fiber, and quality ingredients are replaced with MacroWise snacks loaded with clean protein, nutrients, and natural ingredients. Contents like seed oil, trans-fat, refined flour, processed sugar, corn syrup, high-fructose corn syrup, and artificial sweeteners are replaced with micronutrients, fiber, monk fruit, organic dark chocolate, cacao butter, tapioca fiber, cane sugar, yacon syrup, chocolate liquor, cocoa, cinnamon, vanilla extract, and almond butter.

Instead of eating ultra-processed, nutrient-deficient, unhealthy snacks made with GMOs, soy protein isolate, casein, saturated fat, lactose, gluten, sodium, additives, and preservatives, you get to eat wise-processed, nutrient-dense, healthy snacks enriched with quality protein from natural sources, like hemp, peas, lentils, rice, nuts, seeds, plants, collagen, milk, eggs, fish, chicken, and meat.

Your options for amazing snacks will expand as you transition from one phase to the next. Regardless of which MacroWise phase you're in, this category makes it simple to enjoy your favorite MacroWise snacks while staying in your weight-loss zone.

CHAPTER TWENTY-FOUR

Quick Meals

There are some worthy prepared foods you can utilize to supplement your MacroWise 5 & 1-Thin lifestyle. "Quick Meals" is a category on the list that connects you to a variety of low-sugar items intended to elevate your eating experience and support your weight-loss journey.

The convenient items in this category deliver high-protein, low-carb nutrition without compromising flavor or health. Moving forward, you must find your favorite items for keeping your calorie and macronutrient intake within the correct range. Consuming foods that are not on the list is one of the fastest ways to gain weight without realizing it. Most of the quick meals in the grocery store are high in sugar, calories, carbs, and fat. Eating them will turn a light, macro-wise day into a heavy, macro-dumb lifestyle. This category ensures you have a variety of low-sugar, low-calorie, macro-friendly options for when you need something fast and easy.

During the 90-day, 5 & 1-Thin Phase, you eat 5 MacroWise snacks plus 1 MacroWise meal per day. Essential groceries should always be your go-to source for protein and vegetables when having your meal of the day. Using an air fryer makes it easy to enjoy fresh meals. However, for anyone who doesn't want to shop for fresh groceries or cook, there is another option. There are some decent quick meals you can find in both the refrigerated and frozen sections of the grocery store. These ready-made meals have the right number of calories and macros you need to be satiated. Just heat your MacroWise meal in the microwave and it's ready in minutes with minimal effort.

Some of these fast-food options include creamy garlic chicken with spinach & cauliflower rice, teriyaki beef with mashed cauliflower, lasagna bowl, cauliflower pizza bowl, Korean BBQ-style chicken, beef stroganoff, grilled chicken & broccoli alfredo, fish sticks, chicken nuggets, salmon burgers, crab cakes, cauli mashed braised beef bowl, chicken enchiladas, cheese enchiladas, chili, and more.

We know that the best diet is the one you can stick to long-term. So, even though we don't recommend eating these types of processed meals too often, this option ensures you have everything you need to stay on track. Most of the tasty, quick meals on the list are inexpensive, made with quality ingredients, and reasonably healthy. It's wise to keep some in the freezer as a backup for a rainy day.

Regardless of which MacroWise phase you're in, this category makes it simple to enjoy fast, MacroWise meals while staying in your weight-loss zone.

CHAPTER TWENTY-FIVE

Meal Delivery

There are some quality meal plans you can utilize to simplify your MacroWise 5 & 1-Thin lifestyle. "Meal Delivery" is a category on the list that connects you to a variety of low-sugar items intended to elevate your eating experience and support your weight-loss journey.

The prepared items in this category deliver high-protein, low-carb nutrition, without compromising flavor or health. Moving forward, you must find your favorite items for keeping your calorie and macronutrient intake within the correct range. Consuming foods that are not on the list is one of the fastest ways to gain weight without realizing it. Most of the meals delivered from restaurants are high in sugar, calories, carbs, and fat. Eating them will turn a light, macro-wise day into a heavy, macro-dumb lifestyle. This category ensures you have a variety of low-sugar, low-calorie, macro-friendly options for when you want quality and convenience.

During the 90-day, 5 & 1-Thin Phase, you eat 5 MacroWise snacks plus 1 MacroWise meal per day. Essential groceries should always be your go-to source for protein and vegetables when having your meal of the day. Using an air fryer makes it fast and simple to enjoy fresh meals. However, for anyone who doesn't want to shop for fresh groceries and make their meals from scratch, there is another option. We have vetted several high-quality food companies that deliver fresh, nutrient-dense meals right to your door. Some food companies deliver meal kits with fresh ingredients and recipes for making your own meals. And some ship ready-made meals to warm up with minimal effort. The convenient meals from the food companies on the list taste great and have the right number of calories and macronutrients needed to be satiated.

Meal delivery offers a variety of healthy options to fit any lifestyle choices, including vegan, gluten-free, organic, kosher, grass-fed, and wild-caught protein. Whether you prefer making your meals or simply eating ready-made meals, we have a solution. You can enjoy fresh, tasty foods delivered to your door, like sesame miso salmon with steamed broccoli, citrus-marinated shrimp with squash & mushrooms, chicken teriyaki broccoli bowl, roasted turkey breast with turkey bacon & vegatables, sweet ginger glazed salmon with Bok choy & shiitakes, beef lasagna with cheesy broccoli, and parmesan beef meatballs with spaghetti squash.

Regardless of which MacroWise phase you're in, this category makes it simple to enjoy fast, healthy MacroWise meals while staying in your weight-loss zone. If you're unsure about which meal delivery plan is right for you, ask a MacroWise coach for help.

CHAPTER TWENTY-SIX

Desserts

There are some delicious treats you can utilize to encourage your MacroWise 5 & 1-Thin lifestyle. "Desserts" is a category on the list that connects you to a variety of low-sugar items intended to elevate your eating experience and support your weight-loss journey.

The sweet items in this category deliver natural, high-protein, low-carb nutrition, without compromising flavor or health. Moving forward, you must find your favorite items for keeping your calorie and macronutrient intake within the correct range. Indulging in sweets is one of the fastest ways to gain weight without realizing it. Most of the desserts in the grocery store are either, high in sugar, calories, and carbs, or full of bad chemicals and artificial sweeteners. Consuming them will turn a light macro-wise day into a heavy, macro-dumb lifestyle. This category ensures you have a wide variety of low-sugar, low-calorie, macro-friendly options.

Mainstream desserts made with unhealthy ingredients that leave you craving more are replaced with macro-wise desserts made with healthy ingredients that satisfy. Contents like vegetable & seed oil, high-fructose corn syrup, refined sugar, artificial colors, GMOs, gluten, MSG, synthetic preservatives, and artificial flavors, are replaced with coconut oil, flaxseeds, cocoa butter, fiber, vitamins, minerals, non-GMO, gluten-free, kosher, vegan, and sustainable contents.

There are a variety of delicious desserts on the list you can eat as snacks or enjoy after meals. The healthy items in this category are made with all-natural sweeteners, like monk fruit, organic dark chocolate, cacao butter, tapioca fiber, cane sugar, yacon syrup, chocolate liquor, cocoa, cinnamon, vanilla extract, almond butter, and more. These natural ingredients are used in making some of the world's tastiest foods and are capable of satisfying any sweet tooth. In addition to natural sweeteners, our desserts contain protein that comes from clean, natural sources, like hemp, peas, rice, nuts, seeds, beans, collagen, plants, grass-fed whey, and milk isolate.

You are guaranteed to discover new, healthy favorites on the list that will replace your old, dirty ones. There's a vast selection of chocolate bars, rice crispy treats, ice cream, donuts, cheesecake, brownies, cookies, dark chocolate bites, chocolate-covered nuts, popcorn, cookie dough, pudding, and much more. With MacroWise, you can have your cake and eat it too so long as the cake is from the list.

Regardless of which MacroWise phase you're in, this category makes it simple to enjoy your favorite desserts while staying in your weight-loss zone.

CHAPTER TWENTY-SEVEN

Party Favors

There are some fun items you can utilize to celebrate your MacroWise 5 & 1-Thin lifestyle. "Party Favors" is a unique category on the list that connects you to a variety of feel-good items intended to alter your human experience while supporting your weight-loss journey.

The party items in this category deliver low-calorie, low-carb fun without compromising your body weight or health. Moving forward, you must find your favorite items for keeping your calorie and macronutrient intake within the correct range. Using party treats that are not on the list can be a fast, toxic way to gain weight without realizing it. Most traditional party favors are full of empty calories or have chemicals that lead to binge eating. Using them will turn a clean, macro-wise day into a dirty, macro-dumb lifestyle. This category ensures you have a variety of low-sugar, low-calorie, wise options for when you want to catch a buzz.

MacroWise understands human nature and the need to let loose from time to time. The best diet plan is one that recognizes this reality and plans for it by providing you with safe options. During the 90-day thin phase, it's better to avoid alcohol altogether because the empty calories will kick you out of fat-burning state and make you feel hungry. However, if you stay within your calorie allowance, there are some fun options on the list you can enjoy during this time. Some of those options include beer, wine, hard seltzer, THC-V pills, delta-8 pre-rolls, THC-V & delta-8 vapes, CBD, GABA, kratom, Kanna, muscimol capsules, cigars, and more.

WARNING!! - Be very careful about drinking alcohol! One drink often leads to more and the calories add up fast. Alcohol is considered a macro-nutrient along with protein, carbs, and fat but has no nutritional value to offer. During the first 90 days, there isn't much room in your daily calorie allowance for empty calories from alcohol. You need to make sure that the party materials used do not push you outside of your healthy boundaries. In addition to alcohol, cannabis is a favorite for many but has negative side effects, such as the munchies, which are counterintuitive for losing weight. Unlike regular delta-9 THC derived from cannabis, delta-8 THC derived from hemp provides a lighter high without negative side effects like munchies. Smoking it provides a different effect than ingesting it, but both provide medicinal as well as recreational benefits with little downside.

This category offers you new, macro-wise party favors to replace your old, macro-dumb ones. Having these options makes it easier to stay on track and lose weight.

ABOUT THE AUTHOR

Asher is a weight-loss, fitness, and health coach. He is also the founder of MacroWise, a progressive lifestyle program that helps people lose weight, get fit, and live healthy.

He spent 15 years researching, understanding, and overcoming the complexities of trauma, stress, drug addiction, detox, rehabilitation, sober living, and relapse. He has vast experience working with natural medicines that are known for their exceptional healing properties, some of which are indigenous to foreign countries. He developed an at-home, drug detox kit to help people taper off addictive prescription drugs naturally, such as opioids, benzodiazepines, and sleeping pills. The detox kit was named Attacking Rx, and provided a simple, safe, and natural replacement method for getting off drugs from home.

He applied the crafty lessons learned from overcoming drug addiction towards developing a natural replacement method that helps people lose weight by overcoming sugar and food addiction. This simple method involves eating a variety of low-sugar, nutrient dense foods, 6X a day every 2 1/2 hours from a curated list available at macrowise.com. Ingesting the foods and drinks on the list burns body fat and creates healthy eating habits. He has written 3 books that explain the 3 phases of this progressive lifestyle program called MacroWise. The first book named The Secret to Being Thin, focuses on losing weight. The second book named The Secret to Being Lean, focuses on getting in shape. And the third book named The Secret to Being Healthy, focuses on taking your mental and physical health to the next level. The 3 books are being released to the public in sequential order, at their designated times.

He received his BA from University of Maryland, College Park in 1997, and his master's degree from the school of hard knocks. He spends a lot of his time searching for the highest quality foods, drinks, supplements, and other healthy items, that add value to the list and MacroWise community.

His writings and lectures captivate both wellness experts and layman alike and are enjoyed by people at all levels and from all backgrounds.